Essential Communication Skills for Nursing and Midwifery

Commissioning Editor: Ninette Premdas
Development Editor: Sally Davies
Project Manager: Sruthi Viswam
Designer: Kirsteen Wright
Illustration Manager: Merlyn Harvey
Illustrators: William Le Fever and Cactus

Essential Communication Skills for Nursing and Midwifery

SECOND EDITION

PHILIPPA SULLY
MSc CertEd FPACert RN RM RHV RNT CCRelate
Visiting Lecturer, Reflective Practice, School of Community and Health
Sciences, City University London, UK

JOAN DALLAS
MSc BEd(Hons) PgDip(TA) RN RCNT
Lecturer, Psychology, Communication and Counselling Skills, School of
Community and Health Sciences, City University London, UK

SERIES EDITOR

Maggie Nicol
BSc(Hons) PgDip(Ed) RN
Professor of Clinical Skills, School of Community and Health Sciences,
City University London, UK

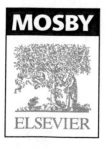

EDINBURGH LONDON NEW YORK OXFORD PHILADELPHIA ST LOUIS SYDNEY TORONTO 2010

MOSBY
ELSEVIER

First edition 2005
Second edition 2010

ISBN 978 0 7234 3527 3

British Library Cataloguing in Publication Data
A catalogue record for this book is available from the British Library

Library of Congress Cataloging in Publication Data
A catalog record for this book is available from the Library of Congress

 your source for books, journals and multimedia in the health sciences

www.elsevierhealth.com

Working together to grow
libraries in developing countries

www.elsevier.com | www.bookaid.org | www.sabre.org

ELSEVIER   BOOK AID International   Sabre Foundation

The Publisher's policy is to use paper manufactured from sustainable forests

Transferred to Digital Printing in 2010

Contents

Preface

Why this book?

Communication underpins everything we do in everyday life as well as in professional practice. What we say, how we say it and what we do communicates a multiplicity of messages. These messages are given and received both consciously and unconsciously.

This book explores how we communicate every day in nursing and midwifery practice. It focuses on the communication skills needed for the development of effective and professional therapeutic relationships. The aim is to enable practitioners to reflect on the effectiveness of their communication skills in practice and to build on their existing skills. This reflection is encouraged, acknowledging that practitioners have differing levels of ability and recognising that these abilities vary according to the situation and the demands made on those involved.

What is it?

Theories offer foundations for exploring the nature of the therapeutic relationship and applying their principles to nursing and midwifery practice. The three theories chosen for this text, humanistic, psychodynamic and systems, acknowledge the importance of both the conscious and unconscious processes that affect our lives and our communication. While we are clear that this is not a book outlining the principles of counselling, we draw on that literature, as well as that of nursing, midwifery, psychology and other relevant sources, to demonstrate the application of effective communication skills to nursing and midwifery practice. These theories of personality and their theoretical principles offer frameworks for explaining and analysing human interactions.

How do I use it?

Each chapter begins with an Introduction and goes on to outline principles underpinning the practice of the skills to be explored. An explanation of the skills is given, followed by a scenario from practice. Specific principles are identified (where appropriate) relating to each scenario as well as the considerations that need to be given to the environment. In this second edition, as well as exploring the specific and sensitive nature of communication in midwifery practice, we have also considered the person with dementia and the specific communication skills that are necessary.

Reflection is integral to the entire text. Readers are invited to consider personal preparation prior to putting a skill into practice. Then, having practised the skill, readers are offered opportunities to reflect on practice. At the end of each scenario, there are reflection-on-practice questions. These are designed to enable readers to analyse their experiences and apply what they have learned to their future practice. If readers have not had a similar experience in practice, they are invited to try and imagine how they would respond if they had.

Each chapter concludes with specific references relevant to the content and in some there are suggestions for further reading. At the end of the book there is a Bibliography to support the theoretical underpinning of the text.

There is a short glossary of specialist terms and an appendix outlining unconscious defences. Other appendices cover obstetric terminology in an emergency and strategies for communication partners of people with aphasia.

We hope that you will find this book interesting, enjoyable and a valuable resource to support and enhance your communications skills and therapeutic relationships.

Philippa Sully
Joan Dallas
London 2010

Acknowledgements

The figures and text below have been reproduced or adapted with permission of the copyright holders and are credited as follows:

Jacobs, M., 2004. Psychodynamic Counselling in Action, 3rd edn. Sage, London, (**Figure 1.1**).

Macmillan, 1996. Professional Relationships: Influences on Health Care. Emap, London, (**Figure 1.3**).

Boud, D., Keogh, R., Walker, D.R., 1985. Reflection: Turning Experience into Learning. Kogan Page, Taylor & Francis, London, (**Figure 2.2**).

Dickson, A., 1982. A Woman in Your Own Right. Quartet, London, (**Figure 6.1**).

Napper, R., Newton, T., 2000. TACTICS. TA Resources, Ipswich, (**Box 9.2**).

Berne, E., 1975. What Do You Say After You Say Hello? Corgi, London, (**Appendix 1: Berne's Ego State Model**).

Gross, R., 2005. Psychology: The Science of Mind and Behaviour, 5th edn. Hodder and Stoughton Educational, London. © 2005 Richard Gross. Reproduced by permission of Hodder & Stoughton Ltd, (**Appendix 2**).

Baron, M., 2009. For permission to reproduce and adapt 'Explaining obstetric terminology in an emergency' from Teaching Notes, with drawings courtesy of M. Laurence (**Appendix 3**).

Simmons-Mackie, N., 2001. Social approaches to aphasia intervention. In: Chapey, R. (Ed.), Language Intervention Strategies in Aphasia and Related Neurogenic Communication Disorders, 4th edn. Lippincott, Williams and Wilkins, Philadelphia, (**Appendix 4**).

We are very grateful to Maurina Baron, Lecturer in Midwifery, London, for her expertise in compiling with us the midwifery content for this edition, and to Jenny Riddell, Consultant Psychotherapist, London, our critical reader.

Introduction

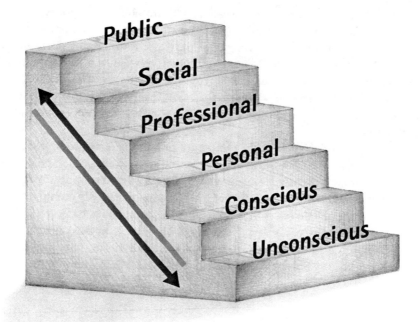

INTRODUCTION

All of us practise skills in communication. Communication skills are transferable across different walks of life and different practice circumstances. Communication is a complex process. It involves a number of interacting factors: (1) physical, e.g. someone with dementia; (2) psychological, e.g. an anxious student and (3) social, e.g. a new mother in her home. How we as practitioners respond in each unique situation requires skilled thought. Effective communication, therefore, requires self-awareness, attention to the unique nature of this episode and a willingness to respond sensitively and flexibly by the use of verbal and non-verbal skills. These skills need to be embodied within the *person* of the practitioner in order for them to respond compassionately and flexibly regardless of the circumstances with which they are faced. Thus, a nurse or midwife does not have to be a specialist in Accident & Emergency (A&E) nursing or neonatal care to demonstrate sensitive communication skills, e.g. how to support a distressed relative.

One model that might be used to understand the process of developing effective communication skills is that developed by Howell (1982), identified in Box 1.1. This model demonstrates how our awareness of our ability changes as we learn new skills and recognize how able, or not, we are to apply them in practice.

For example, the practitioner might not realize how distressing the resuscitation room in A&E might be for the relative and therefore will not offer appropriately sensitive support (**unconscious incompetence**). On the other hand, nurses or midwives may be aware that the resuscitation room is a distressing place for the relative but may not know how to offer adequate support (**conscious incompetence**).

In such situations, **consciously competent** practitioners would be aware of the distressing nature of the environment as well as the needs of the relative. They would therefore consider consciously the best ways to support the relative and choose appropriate interventions. However, **unconsciously competent** practitioners are able to select from a number of observations based on a broad range of experience, about the needs of the relative in this situation. The decision on how to intervene to support the relative is made very quickly: the decision-making process is fast and not necessarily the result of overt

---

Box 1.1 Conscious and unconscious incompetence (Howell 1982)

- Unconscious incompetence
- Conscious incompetence
- Conscious competence
- Unconscious competence.

conscious deliberation. Although it seems ideal for a skilled practitioner to be able to respond in an unconsciously competent way, there are however, practice implications for effective communication. They might be so familiar with their ability that they no longer reflect on their behaviour because it is automatic. This can have a significant and unhelpful interpersonal impact on others, such as failing to explain to the person in their care their intended action or intervention.

CULTURE AND COMMUNICATION

It can be useful to think of culture as being concerned with individuals, groups, organizations, and professions – each have their own assumptions, values and beliefs – and a willingness to be open to those that vary is conducive to promoting cooperative relationships. The relationship may be easier to establish and maintain where there are shared assumptions and beliefs that are linked with shared values. These values in turn produce shared norms that govern patterns of behaviour; according to Egan (2007: 52), 'patterns of behaviour constitute … the bottom line of personal or individual culture'.

'Culture provides each person with specific rules dealing with the universal events of life – birth, mating, childrearing, illness, pain and death' (Munoz & Luckmann 2005: 22). Culture '… is the lens through which we view the world' (Witte & Morrison 1995: 217). A significant task for practitioners therefore is to consider the communication styles and preferences of the people with whom they come into contact, and who may be from a culture that is different from their own. This informed knowledge, however, should not be used to assume that all people from a specific culture would behave in a specific way or require specific considerations; rather it provides the nurse and midwife with options.

Since social rules operate below the level of consciousness, there is also a need for practitioners to increase their awareness with regard to their own behaviour and the cultural factors that influence it. This process can reveal any irrational beliefs, generalizations and stereotypes that they might hold. Practitioners can then reflect on their assumptions and set them aside so they do not interfere with their communication skills. This process of reflection and learning ultimately can lead to increased confidence in communicating effectively.

Throughout this book, the assumption is that readers will come from a wide variety of cultural and ethnic backgrounds. Where appropriate a specific discipline, e.g. nursing or midwifery is identified in the text; where the issue relates to both disciplines, the term 'practitioner' is used.

Individualism and collectivism

Hofstede (1991) used the terms 'individualism' and 'collectivism' to describe the cultural preferences held in relation to the degree to which people considered their needs over those of the group(s) to which they belong. While there will always be variations within any cultural group, western cultures are identified as

Table 1.1 Examples of individualist and collectivist countries and regions (Hofstede 1991)

Individualist	Collectivist
Australia	East and West Africa
Denmark	Hong Kong
New Zealand	Indonesia
UK	Jamaica
USA	Malaysia
	Pakistan
	South America

individualist, where all but the immediate family are placed on the periphery and the individual occupies the central position. A high level of importance is also placed on autonomy, independence and self-assertion (Table 1.1).

In comparison, collectivist cultures are those where family and group membership is central and the individual's life is regulated according to these systems. These cultures operate within an interdependent structure and have a greater desire for the collective rather than focusing on individual achievement (Brown et al 1992). It is important to note that, while a country may be identified as individualist, other cultures within that country may have collectivist trends, for example African-Caribbean, Spanish, or those from the Asian sub-continent in the UK may operate according to their respective ancestries.

Culture, communication and social contexts

Gudykunst (1995) suggests that while individualists and collectivists may belong to the same type of groups (e.g. church, social clubs, a university); the influence that these groups have on the individual is different. One of the areas where these different cultural approaches may be manifest, is in the process of communication and specifically in problem-solving and decision-making. The social context within which the patient/client is seen will also have cultural influence on the communication, for example when entering a client's home, they may ask you to remove your shoes, whereas if they were in hospital this request would not be made.

Those from collectivist cultures were found by Witte & Morrison (1995) to use more accommodating and collaborative strategies when handling conflict and avoided those actions that might lead to animosity, conflict or competition. For example, in Japanese culture, saying 'no' would amount to a 'loss of face' and be experienced as disrespectful; as a consequence Cortazzi & Jin (1997) suggest that more ambiguous statements of disagreement would be used.

Singelis (1994), when comparing individualists with collectivists, found that collectivists, while restricting emotional displays, used more non-verbal and intuitive communication skills and were more indirect in expressing their goals.

This has significant implications in practice when, for example, helping a client manage any pain they may be experiencing, or working collaboratively with the client in goal setting and care planning. Formal rules and procedures were also found to be more important for collectivists than individualists. This would be important for the practitioner to consider when explaining ward restrictions, e.g. no smoking allowed.

Communication across cultures

It is important to remember the key elements of effective communication, since there may be differences when working across cultures. Factors to be considered include the language used and how it is delivered, for example tone of voice, speed of delivery and pronunciation. The consideration of physical characteristics, for example height and body size, also need to be taken into account in order to ensure that neither person feels intimidated. There may be differences across cultures in terms of the appropriateness of touch, preference for personal space, body movements and hand gestures, as well as the use of eye contact.

The factors identified above vary between high- and low-contact cultures; high-contact cultures include Southern Europeans, African and African-Caribbean countries. Northern European and East-Asian cultures are among those representing low-contact cultures. The importance of this relates to what can happen when a person from a high-contact culture meets someone from a low-contact culture and, e.g. offers a handshake that is not reciprocated. The person from the low-contact culture may be perceived as aloof, cold and/or unfriendly. Equally, when a person from a low-contact culture meets someone from a high-contact culture, he or she may find the behaviour of the latter to be intrusive and may also feel that contact has sexual undertones. While humour can have a therapeutic effect, the difference in culture may mean that misunderstanding may ensue, and therefore humour should be used with caution and checks should be made of the patient's/client's understanding.

Self-disclosure
There is a degree of expectation that self-disclosure is part of communication in Western cultures, and this is certainly the case in healthcare practice; this is not however the case, e.g. in African and Japanese cultures. When caring for a patient therefore, practitioners may have to emphasize the importance of clients sharing specific information; however, the practitioners need to be sure that what they are asking the client is necessary and relevant.

These individual differences will also have an impact on the group dynamics, particularly if the members of the team or seminar group have different preferences with regard to self-disclosure. The Johari window is a useful tool for exploring self-disclosure and communication (e.g. Grasha 1995). The facial expressions of people from, e.g. Japanese and Filipino cultures may not portray the uncomfortable emotions they are experiencing: practitioners may therefore have to use their skills to elicit what the person may be feeling and discover how to help. The use of open questions would be appropriate in these circumstances.

Demonstrating respect

Power distance (Hofstede 1991) relates to the degree of equality and respect that is shown to other people, irrespective of place of birth, position, wealth and other social variables. In a number of cultures, establishing and maintaining eye contact with someone who is in a position of authority, or older than the speaker, would be interpreted as insolence and a demonstration of an equality that is misplaced and disrespectful. If the above information is not considered when interacting with people from such cultures, the behaviour of students for example, who use little eye contact when speaking with a ward manager, may be misinterpreted as a lack of interest or a sign that they are aiming to be deceptive. While this may be the case, information will still be needed to support or refute the assumption that is being made.

Values and beliefs

How we relate to others is deeply influenced by our cultural heritage, values and beliefs. Culture is also evident in the development and understanding of psychological theory. Although these theories have evolved in western culture and traditions, they make a significant contribution to our understanding of all people. There is a need to consult the literature and integrate those principles that have been identified as specifically affecting people from diverse cultures. Several authors (e.g. Helman 2007, Kareem & Littlewood 2000, Helms 1999, Munoz & Luckmann 2005) provide informed accounts of these important issues.

An example of a need to ensure integration of relevant perspectives concerns Carl Rogers' explanation of the self-concept (Rogers 1967). In collectivist cultures this may not be so clearly defined, since the self-concept may be closely connected to other people, the groups to which they belong and their roles and relationships in these groups. In individualist cultures, however, the descriptions reflect more of the internal characteristics and those that make the individual unique: for example, 'I am intelligent' in comparison with the collectivist 'I am a mother' (Bochner 1982). In nursing and midwifery practice, this may mean that patients may wish to consult family members and other significant people for advice. They may ask for opinions and direction on decisions that need to be made regarding their health and subsequent treatment. An example might be that pregnant or labouring women from different cultures or faiths would leave the decision-making concerning their care, to their husband, mother or mother-in-law.

PSYCHOLOGICAL THEORIES AND COMMUNICATION

How we see others and ourselves influences how we approach the relationships we make, whether in professional nursing and midwifery practice or in social and intimate situations. *The therapeutic relationship and its development are central to the effectiveness in providing sensitive care.* How practitioners perceive their roles in healthcare delivery, is influenced consciously and unconsciously by their ideas and beliefs about the nature and lives of people and the context within which care is offered.

Theories of personality provide a psychological as well as a philosophical framework by which we can consider our interactions with other people. Three psychological approaches are used to inform this text. These are: (1) humanistic theory, drawing on the work of Maslow (1954) and Rogers (1967); (2) psychodynamic theory, e.g. the work of Freud (see also Jacobs 2004, Bowlby 1988 and Winnicott 1965); and (3) systems theory, e.g. the works of Huffington et al (2004), Hinschelwood & Skogstad (2000), Menzies Lyth (1959/1988), Obholzer & Roberts (1994) and Roberts (1994). Psychodynamic and systems theories can be seen to interlink, offering perceptions on individual and group processes in teams and organizations.

Theories provide us with an understanding of those factors that enhance or detract from our personal and psychological development. Although nursing and midwifery are patient- and client-centred, the person of the patient or client may be forgotten, e.g. when the daily completion of pre-printed care plans is carried out without consultation with those in our care. However, Stiles et al (1986) confirm that it is the **relationship** that is the significant feature in any effective encounter. The relationship and the core qualities required to establish it form the basis of person-centred theory and are explored in great depth by Rogers (1967) and later by Mearns & Thorne (2007).

Psychological theories offer foundations for exploring the nature of the therapeutic relationship and applying their principles to professional practice. There is also acknowledgement of the importance of both the conscious and unconscious psychological processes that affect our lives and our communication.

Humanistic perspective

Therapeutic nursing and midwifery interventions need to be based on sound psychological principles, although practitioners are often unaware of these as they carry out their daily work. Principles of cognitive-behavioural therapy are being used, e.g. when encouraging a patient who is undergoing a stressful or unpleasant procedure to take deep breaths or imagine a pleasant scene, sound or smell. The various psychological perspectives and their principles are succinctly outlined in Palmer (2000), and, depending on the specific area of practice, one perspective may be used more than another. For example, in mental health nursing a therapeutic group might be based on psychodynamic principles.

The humanistic perspective is seen as the third force in psychology after psychodynamic and behavioural theories. Two theories that come under the humanistic umbrella are person-centred theory and transactional analysis. The following section will provide a brief overview of these perspectives and their application to nursing and midwifery practice.

Person-centred theory (Carl Rogers)
Humanistic models acknowledge the influence of childhood and current experiences on life and that these experiences are significant in enabling change,

leading to a greater sense of wellbeing. Maslow (1954) and Rogers (1967) shared the belief that individuals are motivated to achieve their potential. Rogers explored the development of the self-concept and the conditions of worth that individuals develop during their early years, which often prevented them reaching their potential in adult life. Conditions of worth are introjections, i.e. pieces of information from adult figures and experiences that children record and believe to be true, until they form part of their thinking about themselves. While these introjections may have a positive influence on the individual's self-esteem, this is not always the case, e.g. people being told over considerable time, that they are not important, will believe it. In nursing and midwifery, this may present where a patient may not ask for assistance or pain relief because they feel they do not deserve it, since they are not as ill or as distressed as the next person.

This gap between real self and ideal self may become even wider, where illness or the individual's health changes their real or perceived body image, e.g. in pregnancy or someone with Parkinson's disease.

In 1967, Rogers developed the person-centred theory and based this on his notion of the therapeutic relationship: 'Good communication ... within or between men, is always therapeutic' (Rogers 1967: 330). He identified three factors (the core conditions) necessary in the psychological environment for personal growth: genuineness, showing acceptance and empathizing. Like most authors at the time, Rogers used only the masculine noun, but in his later works he used inclusive language.

Genuineness/congruence

According to Rogers (1967: 33), being genuine 'involves the willingness to be and to express in my words and behaviour, the various feelings and attitudes which exist in me ... it is only by providing the genuine reality which is in me that the other person can successfully seek for the reality in him'. This does not give one person the authority to reveal all that one feels and thinks without considering the impact it might have on the other person. It does however, invite practitioners to pay attention to their thoughts, feelings and behaviours and consider what these are telling them about themselves, the patient and the situation. It also enables practitioners to reveal what would be felt as most beneficial and relevant in a respectful and sensitive manner.

Acceptance

'By acceptance I mean a warm regard for him as a person of unconditional self-worth, of value no matter what his condition, his behaviour or his feelings' (Rogers 1967: 34). Rogers identifies the importance of being able to *experience* this acceptance in the relationship. An essential skill in nursing and midwifery is being able to respond immediately in an accepting way, even if the client, for some reason is unable to receive what you offer. It is important to be aware of what the effect of this might be, so the practitioner does not respond inappropriately, such as being defensive. This approach is also known as 'unconditional positive regard' (Rogers 1967).

Empathy

Empathy is the ability to 'feel a continuing desire to understand ... the client's feelings and communications as they seem to him at that moment'. Rogers identifies this as 'a deep empathic understanding' (Rogers 1967: 34).

Rogers clarifies this as an understanding **with** not **about** the other person: 'Real communication occurs ... when we listen with understanding' (Rogers 1967: 331). Rogers admits that he was not always able to achieve these qualities in the relationship and cautions that the other person may not always be able to accept this type of relationship. It would be worth exploring those situations, patient groups, age dimensions or illness categories where you find it difficult to offer the above qualities.

It may be appropriate to disclose something personal related to the situation in order to demonstrate empathy; however it is *imperative* that this disclosure is for the benefit of the client rather than a reaction by the practitioner to a situation they, personally, are finding difficult. *Skilled* self-disclosure is about supporting the client's experience rather than about being dismissive of or devaluing it.

As a nurse or midwife, it may be discouraging if you feel that you have offered your best to a client and/or their family and they have not shown signs of appreciation or responded to what you have offered. Although we all need to feel a sense of achievement, it must be remembered that the practitioner–client relationship is not a reciprocal one; therefore the depth of appreciation that is desired from the client may be unreasonable. It is for this reason that practitioners need to ensure that their own support systems are robust and varied enough to meet their psychological needs. This includes support from, e.g. friends, colleagues, and clinical supervision.

Transactional analysis (Eric Berne)

Transactional analysis is a theory of personality, child development, social psychology and psychopathology. Eric Berne left his psychodynamic background and developed this theory, which continues to be refined and developed. The theory is used extensively in clinical, organizational and educational fields and is placed under the humanistic umbrella.

The philosophical assumptions underpinning transactional analysis are that people are 'OK', i.e. one human being unconditionally accepts another, and that change is possible (See Appendix 1). There is also a belief that, unless a person has very severe learning difficulties (and this view is debatable), people are capable of learning to take responsibility for their decisions and actions. The principles of transactional analysis that have been drawn upon and applied in this book are those of 'OKness' and 'contracting' (Stewart 2007). These are based on the belief that as human beings, we are all worthy of respect. The process of contracting therefore enables people to negotiate agreements and expectations of one another from a position of mutual respect, and is an essential part of care planning. These principles are more explicit in Chapter 6, yet they also apply to other sections of the book. The analysis of transactions using the ego state model appears mainly in Chapter 6.

Psychodynamic perspectives

Alongside the schools of thought offered by the humanistic (discussed above) and systems (discussed below) perspectives, we address the contributions of psychodynamic theories, in that they recognize both the conscious and unconscious psychological processes manifest in our interactions with others and with ourselves. Psychodynamic theory of personality provides explanations of how we relate to ourselves and our inner worlds, as well as how we relate to others and the outside world. This outline is not intended to be exhaustive, but rather to provide an overview of the relevant aspects of the theory in relation to this text on communication in nursing and midwifery practice. (For broader explorations of psychodynamic theories and the views of different theorists, a Bibliography is offered at the end of the book.)

Psychodynamic views of the human psyche are based on the view that our psyche (mind/emotions/spirit/self) is active (Jacobs 2004: 6). Sigmund Freud (Maddi 1989) described this as a psychosocial conflict between our instinctive motivation ('id'), our conscience (superego – the seat of our 'values and taboos which are learnt from society') and our ego or conscious sense of who we are, which develops from the id (Maddi 1989: 627).

Different theorists have differing perspectives on the structure and 'internal relationships' (Jacobs 2004: 8) of our psyche, as well as on the nature of our motivation and psychic conflict. What they have in common is the view that our psyche relates to the outside world and others in it, *as well as* to our own inner worlds and aspects of ourselves. They also recognize the different levels of awareness of the psyche and how these are manifest in our behaviour, the manner in which we relate to ourselves and to others, and thus in the ways in which we communicate.

Our inner aspects of ourselves develop as a consequence of our early relationships with significant others, especially our primary carers. These real relationships have their corresponding inner images or objects, which develop throughout childhood and remain active within our psyche. Jacobs (2004: 8) points out that: 'we can just as easily love, hate, criticize or fear parts of ourselves as we can other people'. These theories offer perspectives, therefore, on how we relate to ourselves as well as to other people.

Different psychodynamic theorists have different ideas as to what motivates us to behave as we do. However, there is general agreement among them that in order to reduce or avoid the anxiety caused by psychic conflict, e.g. having to choose between what we feel we **ought** to do and what we **want** to do in circumstances that are emotionally demanding, we might deny that the dilemma exists and thus avoid addressing it.

Conflict

Bateman et al (2000: 50) describe the nature of the conflict according to Freud as being: 'between the present and the past and between culture and instinct … between the outer world or external reality and our inner world or psychic reality'. Maddi (1989: 640) describes Jung's theory of conflict as being between the '*ego* (or conscious, individualistic mind)' and 'the *personal unconscious* (formed of socially unacceptable mental content that was once conscious but has been forced out of awareness by defences)' (original italics). Winnicott (1965) described the conflict as being between our needs and the need to please others, which in extreme cases can lead to the development of a false self. He describes the false self as 'this false front being a defence designed to protect the true self' (Winnicott 1986: 33). It develops when the true self needs protection from being traumatized or severely wounded again.

Unconscious defences

In order to deal with aspects of ourselves which, if experienced consciously, might cause 'unbearable anxiety or psychic pain' (Bateman et al 2000: 21), we use **unconscious defences**. These include denial, repression, projection, reaction formation, rationalization, conversion and psychosomatic reactions, regression, phobic avoidance, depersonalization and confusion, sublimation and displacement. (For an extensive description of these, see Gross 2005, Ch. 42 and Bateman et al 2000, Part 1.) (See also Appendix 2 in this volume.)

Transference relationship

What is significant about our past experiences is their presentation in the present. This is clearly evident in the nature of the **transference relationship** where we relate unconsciously to others in the here-and-now as we would have related to other people with whom we had important relationships in the past. Healthcare practitioners, because they work with people who are frequently in physically and/or emotionally dependent relationships with them, may be at the receiving end of strong transferences. This can arise because of their relative position of power in relation to the dependency needs of those in their care, and the emotions from the past that this evokes in their patients and clients. Practitioners' personal experiences, e.g. as parents or patients can colour their perceptions of those in their care and thus have a significant impact on their styles of communication with them. An example would be practitioners who have been survivors of domestic violence or have experienced a neonatal death, and who may **not** be aware that their responses to the client are inappropriately manifest.

It is important therefore for practitioners to be aware of this so they do not find themselves responding to the transference, rather than to the needs of those they are caring for in that specific moment, thereby fulfilling the unconscious role in which the patient or client sees them, i.e. acting out the **counter-transference relationship**, and fulfilling the patient's/client's expectations from the past. How they respond to us can inform us about what we might represent for them at an unconscious level. Awareness of this can help us to respond empathetically to how they are feeling in the here-and-now. For example, if in past relationships the person has been silent and submissive, they will also be silent and submissive in their relationship of dependence with you; not expecting to have any choice in their care (transference). You respond unconsciously by not offering them any choice in their care (counter-transference). On **reflection**, you recognize your response as unusual for you and realize the need to change how you relate to that person.

Insight and reflection

Freud defined the mental activity that was not conscious but readily could be brought into consciousness as the preconscious, 'such as a memory of a fact, a feeling or an event, fact or feeling' (Jacobs 2004: 11). Nelson-Jones (2001: 27) describes it as:

> Consist(ing) of everything that can easily exchange the unconscious state for the conscious one. Thus the preconscious is latent and capable of becoming conscious, while the unconscious is repressed and is unlikely to become conscious without great difficulty ... (It) may be viewed as a screen between the unconscious and consciousness ...

This *preconscious awareness* is therefore an aspect of our ego that is out of awareness but can be retrieved through reflection.

The *Reflection on practice* sections in each chapter aim to enable practitioners to gain access to those aspects of their work that were out of awareness at the time, but which can be retrieved through reflection-on-action by reviewing their work in a structured manner (see Boud et al's 1985 *Model of Reflection*, Ch. 2).

Figure 1.1 illustrates the triangle of insight, as described by Jacobs (2004: 139). The significance of this triangle is that patients and clients might respond to nurses and midwives as if they are significant people from their past. Likewise, they might employ unconscious defences to deal with distressing situations in similar ways to those they have used in earlier stages of development. Indeed, this process of the past being manifest in present interactions can occur in relationships other than those between practitioners and clients, e.g. it can happen in the supervisory relationship between practitioner and supervisor (Hawkins & Shohet 2006: Ch. 7).

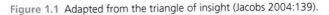

Present-in-here
Counsellor
(nurse, midwife) client

Past-back-then
Parent–child

Present-out-there
Client (patient)–other

Figure 1.1 Adapted from the triangle of insight (Jacobs 2004:139).

If as practitioners we can be sensitive to this process, we can learn much about how to respond appropriately and empathetically to those in our care, and learn more about our other professional relationships and practice through mentorship, supervision and reflection (see Ch. 2).

Johari window

The different levels of communication, and indeed our understanding of how people present themselves in everyday relationships, are evident in the description of our psychic awareness described by the Johari window (Fig. 1.2). The four areas of the Johari window **relate to different aspects of ourselves**. These aspects will influence our levels of communication and our understanding of how other people, as well as we ourselves, behave.

The 'public self' is that part of ourselves which we acknowledge and which others can see; the 'private self' is that part of ourselves which we acknowledge but do not disclose to others. The 'unconscious self' is unknown to ourselves and others, but the 'blind self' could be described as those aspects of ourselves that we deny, because if we did not do so we would experience threatening emotions and consequently anxiety. This denial is an unconscious defence (see Appendix 2). Others might see aspects of ourselves of which we are unaware, i.e. the 'blind self' and interpret our behaviour with this in mind. Each area of the Johari window has an impact on the others; an example is that if the 'hidden self' is large, the remaining areas are proportionately smaller. A large 'hidden' (or private) section will reflect the style of communication used and may, for example, lead to tension in a group. This individual is likely to be less available or open to feedback. In contrast, where the 'public area' is appropriately available to others, the

	Known to self	Not known to self
Known to others	**Open area** (our 'public self': the person we ourselves and others see)	**Blind area** (our 'blind self': aspects of ourselves others can see but we cannot) This aspect is reduced by being open to feedback
Not known to others	**Hidden area** (our 'private self': aspects of ourselves we are aware of but choose not to disclose to others) This aspect is reduced by self-disclosure.	**Unknown area** ('unconscious self': unknown to others and to ourselves)

Figure 1.2 Johari window (adapted from Luft 1969).

communication experience is fluent. It is also appreciated that the **context** and the **nature of the relationship** that person is in, will influence how they communicate. The Johari window can therefore be seen as a dynamic – as opposed to a static – model, to help appreciate patterns of communication as well as a framework by which to understand self-awareness.

Systems perspectives

As practitioners, we do not exist in isolation. Systems perspectives address the nature of our roles in groups, organizations and families. An open system is one that has an external boundary through which it takes 'inputs'. Within this boundary, systems of activities occur which convert or transform (Armstrong 2005) the input through 'the inputs to outputs' (Roberts 1994: 28). The external boundary separates the organization from the external environment, but it needs to be permeable enough to manage exchanges between the external and internal environments so that the primary task of the organization can be achieved. An example would be the manager of a community nursing team ensuring that district nurses are supported in their roles of delivering nursing care (the task of the service) when there is pressure on them also to run errands such as collect shopping because there is a shortage of home helps in the local social services department. The manager would manage the boundary between the nursing service and the social service by addressing the problem with the managers in social services.

A key concept in this approach to describing and understanding what goes on in organizations is that of interaction and interrelatedness (Armstrong 2005, Arnold et al 1998). A fundamental tenet therefore of systems theory is that the whole is greater than the sum of its parts, and the 'qualities of an open, ongoing system are emergent out of the interaction of its parts' (Broderick 1993: 38). Thus patterns of behaviour and communication become evident in the processes of working in groups and teams. Individuals in a group or team, however, bring their own conscious and unconscious motives to the task of the organization (Roberts 1994). Some theorists in this field are Armstrong (2005), Menzies Lyth (1959/1988), Obholzer & Roberts (1994), Roberts (1994) and Skogstad (2000).

Groups
How we behave in groups serves both a conscious and an unconscious function for the group as well as the organization in which we work (Armstrong 2005, Obholzer & Roberts 1994). How we interact with those with whom we work, including with those in our care, is not only related to our own conscious and unconscious processes and those of our patients and clients, but it is also related to how we see ourselves and our practice in relation to the primary task of the organizations in which we work (Hinschelwood & Skogstad 2000). These authors point out that in organizations, there are '*unconscious* assumptions, attitudes and beliefs about the work task and how to perform it' (Hinschelwood & Skogstad 2000: 9; original italics). This shared culture results in systems of behaviour in groups and subgroups within the organization, such as taking on particular roles,

sharing unconscious defences and even maintaining particular working practices, whether effective or not. An example of this is what Street (1995) calls 'the tyranny of niceness' in nursing culture, where nurses perceive their roles as always having to be nice. This means that often they do not feel able to acknowledge and/or express 'unacceptable' feelings appropriately, such as impatience or anger. This culture of niceness can be disempowering as well as oppressive.

Caring for people in distress or at major transitions in their lives, is emotionally demanding and anxiety provoking. Consequently, as individuals and as groups, we develop ways of defending ourselves from the emotional stress and anxiety this engenders (Menzies Lyth 1959/1988, Obholzer & Roberts 1994). In order that we do not lose sight of our part in the delivery of care, it is important that we try to stay in touch with how we **understand** our roles as nurses or midwives in the organization, as well as keeping in touch with our feelings about our work. This will help us to avoid being unconsciously sucked 'into performing a function on behalf of others' (Obholzer & Roberts 1994: 131), i.e. acting out roles unconsciously assigned to us, and accepted by us, by the groups or teams in which we practice. An example of this would be a group member who always seems to be relied upon to become angry in meetings, unconsciously expressing the frustration and anger of all the team members (Obholzer & Roberts 1994, Ch. 14) (see also Ch. 9 in this volume).

Systems perspectives provide us with explanations for the interactions between individuals, groups and teams – both conscious and unconscious – in the organizational contexts of professional practice. It is important that, as far as possible, we are aware of these processes and how they might affect the ways in which people, including ourselves, behave in order that we communicate sensitively and effectively in professional practice.

MODEL OF COMMUNICATION

The model of communication chosen to underpin the text (Fig. 1.3) illustrates that not all **intentions** for **interactions** with others are conscious. It puts each interaction within the wider context both within the individuals involved and within the environment in which it takes place. It addresses the view that communication is on a **number of levels**. Each of us brings a personal as well as a social history to each interaction and these interactions have both conscious and unconscious antecedents and consequences. Psychodynamic theory recognizes 'the different layers of understanding' (Jacobs 2004: 14–16) inherent in communication with others. These possible differences in meaning are identified below.

Each interaction is preceded by the individual's personal **history**. These histories are rooted in personal experience, which are conscious and unconscious. How people **interpret** experiences is grounded in their cultural and personal heritage. Each person involved in the interaction approaches it with an **intention**, which is either conscious and/or unconscious. The intention sets an agenda for the desired **consequences** of the **interaction**.

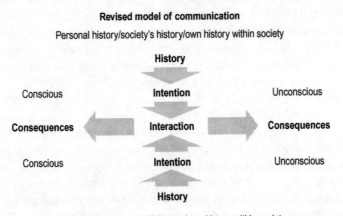

Revised model of communication

Personal history/society's history/own history within society

Figure 1.3 Model of communication (Macmillan 1996).

These **consequences** are both conscious and unconscious. An unconscious consequence may be that a nurse involved in the interaction may become very irritated with a patient. As nurses, we may not be aware that we are irritated, since being irritated with those in our care is not felt to be an acceptable response to a patient, either professionally or culturally. Despite this, we may be aware that our tone of voice has become harsh and raised. Reflecting on our communication and unusually raised tone, we may discover that this was a **consequence** of our feelings of irritation of which we were not aware.

In the same communication, the process, e.g. of the patient's or client's **interaction** with the practitioner, is influenced by their personal experiences in their past and current **history**, both conscious and unconscious, of being in a position of possible dependency; a perceived role in some cultures of a service user. These feelings might evoke earlier experiences of being dependent and perhaps out of control of the situation they are in. The **consequences** could be that the patient or client responds defensively or submissively, leaving the practitioner confused as to the needs of the person to whom they offer care.

CONCLUSION

This volume is a 'how-to' book. As such, it does not claim to be definitive, but to provide readers with frameworks with which to review and develop their communication skills. As effective communication is fundamental to all nursing and midwifery practice, we hope it offers practitioners the opportunity to reflect on as well as to value their communication skills, in turn enabling them to communicate sensitively and confidently throughout their professional lives.

References

Armstrong, D., 2005. Organization in the Mind: Psychoanalysis, Group Relations and Organizational Consultancy. Karnac, London.

Arnold, J., Cooper, C.L., Robertson, I.T., 1998. Work Psychology: Understanding Human Behaviour in the Workplace, 3rd edn. *Financial Times*/Pitman Publishing, London.

Bateman, A., Brown, D., Pedder, J., 2000. Introduction to Psychotherapy: an Outline of Psychodynamic Principles and Practice, 3rd edn. Routledge, Hove.

Bochner, S., (Ed.), 1982. Cultures in Contact: Studies in Cross-Cultural Interaction. Pergamon Press, Oxford.

Boud, D., Keogh, R., Walker, D.R., 1985. Reflection: Turning Experience Into Learning. Kogan Page, London.

Bowlby, J., 1988. A Secure Base. Routledge, London.

Broderick, C.B., 1993. Understanding Family Process Basics of Family Systems Theory. Sage, London.

Brown, D., Brown, R., Hinkle, S., Ely, P., Fox-Cardomone, L., Maras, P., Taylor, L., 1992. Recognising group diversity: individualist-collectivist and autonomous related social orientations and their implications for intergroup processes. British Journal of Social Psychology 31, 327–342.

Cortazzi, M., Jin, T.L., 1997. Communication for learning across cultures. In: McNamara, D., Harris, R. (Eds.), Overseas Students in Higher Education. Routledge, London.

Egan, G., 2007. The Skilled Helper: A Problem-Management and Opportunity-Development Approach to Helping, 8th edn. Brooks/Cole, Pacific Grove.

Grasha, A., 1995. Practical Applications of Psychology, 4th edn. Harper Collins, New York.

Gross, R.D., 2005. Psychology: the Science of Mind and Behaviour, 5th edn. Hodder and Stoughton, London.

Gudykunst, W., 1995. Anxiety/uncertainty management (AUM) theory. In: Wiseman, R. (Ed.), Intercultural Communication Theory. Sage, London.

Hawkins, P., Shohet, R., (Eds.), 2006. The seven-eyed supervision: a process model. In: Supervision in the Helping Professions. Open University Press, Maidenhead.

Helman, C., 2007. Culture, Health and Illness, 5th edn. Hodder Arnold, London.

Helms, J., 1999. Black and White Racial Identity: Theory, Research and Practice. Praeger, Conn.

Hinschelwood, R.D., Skogstad, W., 2000. Observing Organisations. Anxiety, Defence and Culture in Health Care. Routledge, London.

Hofstede, G., 1991. Cultures and Organisations: Intercultural Co-operation and Its Importance for Survival. Harper Collins, London.

Howell, W., 1982. The Empathic Communicator. Wadsworth, Pacific Grove.

Huffington, C., Armstrong, D., Halton, W., Hoyle, L., Pooley, J., (Eds.), 2004. Working Below the Surface The Emotional Life of Organizations. Karnac, London.

Jacobs, M., 2004. Psychodynamic Counselling in Action, 3rd edn. Sage, London.

Kareem, J., Littlewood, K. (Eds.), 2000. Intercultural Therapy, Blackwell Science, London.

Luft, J., 1969. Of Human Interaction. National Press, Palo Alto.

Macmillan, 1996. Professional Relationships: Influences on Health Care. Emap, London.

Maddi, S.R., 1989. Personality Theories: a Comparative Analysis, 5th edn. Wadsworth, Pacific Grove.

Maslow, A., 1954. Motivation and Personality. Harper Row, London.

Mearns, D., Thorne, B., 2007. Person-Centred Approaches to Counselling Psychology, 3rd edn. Sage, London.

Menzies Lyth, I.E.P., 1959/1988. The functioning of social systems as a defence against anxiety: a report on a study on the nursing service of a general hospital. Reprinted in Menzies Lyth, I.E.P. (1988) Containing Anxiety in Institutions: Selected Essays. Free Association Books, London, pp. 43–85.

Munoz, C., Luckmann, J., 2005. Transcultural Communication in Nursing. Thomson Learning, London.

Nelson-Jones, R., 2001. Theory and Practice of Counselling and Therapy, 3rd edn. Sage, London.

Obholzer, A., Roberts, V.Z., 1994. The troublesome individual and the troubled institution. In: Obholzer, A., Roberts, V.Z. (Eds.), The Unconscious at Work: Individual and Organizational Stress in the Human Services. Routledge, London.

Palmer, S. (Ed.), 2000. Introduction to Counselling and Psychotherapy. Sage, London.

Roberts, V.Z., 1994. The organization of work: contributions from open systems theory. In: Obholzer, A., Roberts, V.Z. (Eds.), The Unconscious at Work: Individual and Organizational Stress in the Human Services. Routledge, London.

Rogers, C., 1967. On Becoming a Person: a Therapist's View of Psychotherapy. Constable, London.

Singelis, T., 1994. Bridging the gap between culture and communication. In: Bouvy, A.M., Van de Vijver, F., Boski, P., Schmitz, P. (Eds.), Journeys into Cross-cultural Psychology. Swets & Zeitlinger, Lisse.

Skogstad, W., 2000. Working in a world of bodies: a medical ward. In: Hinshelwood, R.D., Skogstad, W. (Eds.), Observing Organisations. Routledge, London.

Stewart, I., 2007. Transactional Analysis Counselling in Action, 3rd edn. Sage, London.

Stiles, W.B., Shapiro, D.A., Elliot, E., 1986. Are all psychotherapies equivalent? Am. Psychol. 41 (2), 165–180.

Street, A., 1995. Nursing Replay. Churchill Livingstone, Melbourne.

Winnicott, D.W., 1986. Home is Where We Start From. Harmondsworth, Penguin.

Winnicott, D.W. (Ed.), 1965. Ego distortion in terms of the true and false self. In: The Maturational Processes and the Facilitating Environment. Hogarth Press, London.

Witte, K., Morrison, K., 1995. Intercultural and cross cultural health communication: understanding people and motivating healthy behaviours. In: Wiseman, R. (Ed.), Intercultural Communication Theory. Sage, London.

Further reading on cultural issues and professional practice

Giger, J., Davidhizar, R., 2008. Transcultural Nursing: Assessment and Intervention. Mosby Elsevier, St Louis.

Owusu-Bempah, K., Howitt, D., 2000. Psychology Beyond Western Perspectives. British Psychological Society, Leicester.

Perez, M., Luquis, R., 2008. Cultural Competence in Health Education and Health Promotion. Jossey-Bass, San Francisco.

Spector, R., 2008. Cultural Diversity in Health and Illness. Pearson, Warwick.

Further reading on psychodynamic theory

Bateman, A., Brown, D., Pedder, J., 2000. Introduction to Psychotherapy: An Outline of Psychodynamic Principles and Practice, 3rd edn. Routledge, Hove.

Malan, D.H., 1995. Individual Psychotherapy and the Science of Psychodynamics, 2nd edn. Hodder Arnold, London.

2

Reflecting on practice

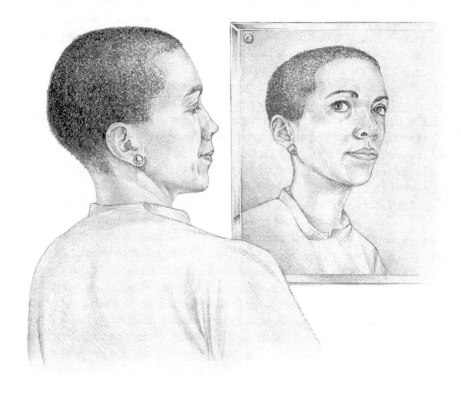

INTRODUCTION

A wealth of untapped knowledge is embedded in the practices and the 'know how'
of expert nurse clinicians, but this knowledge will not expand or fully develop
unless nurses systematically record what they learn from experience ... There is
much to learn and appreciate as practising nurses uncover meanings acquired as a
result of helping, coaching and intervening in the significantly human events that
comprise the art and science of nursing.

(Benner 2001: 11)

Practitioners' ability to reflect on practice is fundamental to their development
as sound, creative and responsive professionals. Their ability to transform their
practice through the processes of reviewing their inner experiences of their work
and relating them to the outer realities, e.g. contextual and interpersonal, of
their experiences, takes courage and a willingness to be open to new ideas and
perspectives. The capacity to reflect upon and transform practice of necessity
therefore takes into account practitioners' *feelings* as well as their thoughts. Johns
(2005: 2) describes reflection as a process that is both subjective and particular.
It is a fusion of sensing, perceiving, intuiting and thinking related to a specific
experience in order to develop insights into self and practice.

Reflective practice therefore has a purpose; its aim is to promote actions that
transform individuals' practice so they resolve dilemmas or contradictions, build
on their strengths and so offer more insightful and sensitive care. It also assumes
that the practitioner has an image of the nature of sound practice and how they
want to develop their skills to attain this.

The processes of reflection that can promote the development of the person
of the practitioner, and thus the transformation of their work, address the
feelings that their experiences elicit. Reflection is also context bound. What we
experience in one situation may be very different emotionally from another,
although outwardly the issues brought to us by people needing our care, may seem
similar. When thinking of models of reflection, it is clear that reflective practice
is more than considering our overt observation of external signs of situations,
environments and our demonstrable responses. It is also about being aware of
our inner processes as we respond to these observations. These inner processes are
crucial components of our abilities to interpret what we perceive and how we offer
our skills in any given situation. What were we feeling when we were introduced
to a woman attending her first antenatal clinic? How did we experience the
atmosphere in a home when we were offering care to a family's older relation?

Reflection also allows for attentive listening for triggers that are not directly
attributed to the recognized five senses, as it also recognizes the 'sixth' sense, which
could be called 'intuition'.

It is through the process of reflection on what we feel, that will offer us clues
to what we might have perceived but about which we were not consciously aware,
i.e. tacit understanding. In this way we can gain further insight into our inner

processes that, in turn, can inform us about our skills at all levels; thus we can develop both professionally and personally. When we take time to reflect, we are creating opportunities for ourselves to make connections between our experiences as *people*, in a variety of professional situations that link personal practice, theory and research, and consequently, we can transform our delivery of nursing and midwifery care. The reflective process has a direct impact on the decisions we make about our professional practice, how we implement and evaluate them. Awareness, therefore, of our inner processes, how we reflect-in and -on-action and the contexts of our relationships that are part of everyday practice, enables us to develop further our skills in emotional intelligence – intelligence that is central to every aspect of our lives. Self-awareness, a vital component of emotional intelligence (e.g. Golman 1998) (see also Ch. 4 in this volume), is crucial to our sensitivity as professional practitioners who work with people who need our services.

Reflection also allows for the structured exploration of the knowledge, skills, attitudes and perceptions – tacit and overt – that underpin professional practice. It also lays the foundation for the continuing professional development required by the Nursing and Midwifery Council (2008a) and lifelong learning.

To enable you to develop your skills of reflection, sections on Reflection on practice are included in each chapter. These are designed to provide you with a framework for thinking about your professional practice and what you might learn from your experiences at all levels. They are not intended to be definitive.

THE REFLECTIVE PROCESS

Benner (2001) and Schön (1991) in different ways, describe the reflective process as involving:

- **Action**, which may not necessarily include overt thought, as sometimes we respond to the immediacy of a situation, e.g. in an emergency where we respond reflexively but perceptively
- **Critical thought**, which includes the processes of seeking reasons for our interpretations of experiences and behaviour that enable us to evaluate and make judgements
- **The self**: when we have an experience, we also have a sense of ourselves in that situation. Any interpretation we make will give the process or experience meaning that is personal to ourselves. Meaning therefore is personal and involves us completely, both consciously and unconsciously, and includes thoughts, feelings, frames of reference, values and attitudes. Many of these perceptions are tacit, but can be reviewed when we reflect on our practice.

Reflection therefore engages all of our feelings, thoughts and behaviour, i.e. it is not solely a detached exercise in thinking (Fig. 2.1).

Where reflection is based on and in particular episodes or aspects of practice, it enables practitioners to ground their thoughts and feelings and keep the

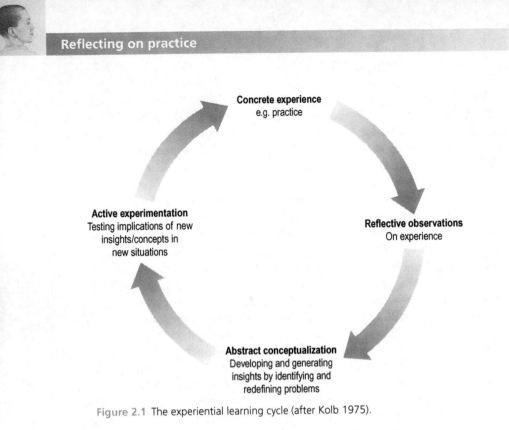

Concrete experience
e.g. practice

Reflective observations
On experience

Abstract conceptualization
Developing and generating
insights by identifying and
redefining problems

Active experimentation
Testing implications of new
insights/concepts in
new situations

Figure 2.1 The experiential learning cycle (after Kolb 1975).

reflection focused. This helps to prevent reflection from becoming a circular and nebulous process where nothing changes or, at worst, where it becomes a means of negative criticism, leading to paralysis of thought and action.

There are a number of models of reflection in the literature. Benner (2001: 2) explores the difference between **knowing how** and **knowing that**. Reflective practice helps us to **know how**. This occurs when we reflect **on** our actions (after the event) having reflected **in** action during the event (Schön 1991). Schön (1991) also describes professionals' **reflection-in-action** as the capacity to vary their practice so they respond appropriately to situations *as they occur*. This process enables practitioners to provide flexible and sensitive care without stopping in the middle of an event in order to review how to respond. **Reflection-on-action** is what occurs after the event and enables the practitioner to learn from experiences of all sorts, not solely those that have been particularly problematic or exceptionally novel. Kolb (1975) however, describes this reflection-on-action as the cycle of learning from experience (Fig. 2.1).

The capacity to learn from positive experiences, however, is also important, as it enables us to identify processes and skills that are sound and can be used more widely in other situations. These positive responses can help us to become more confident in our abilities, while recognizing that we need to keep an open mind about the potential value and application of our established skills and how they can promote new learning.

This model (Fig. 2.1) enables us to think about the processes that enable us to learn from experience. It is also worth considering what we anticipate from new experiences ahead – **anticipatory reflection** (Sully et al 2008, Wilson 2008, van Manen 1991). What we identify about our preconceptions about the future event and the emotions these elicit, can raise our awareness of how our inner processes might affect our **concrete experience** in the realities of practice, our reflective observations on these experiences, and how we might translate these perceptions into **abstract concepts**. We can then try out these new insights in other situations by **active experimentation**. An anticipatory reflection is illustrated in Box 2.1, i.e. it illustrates the process of reflecting on an experience that lies ahead.

Your experiences of people with mental illness whom you have met in other walks of life may influence how you perceive this placement. You may find that you are quite apprehensive about working with people whose illnesses are evident more in their behaviour and manner of relating, rather than in physical manifestations. Perhaps this is because you anticipate that they will react in unpredictable ways, or you may feel unable to help in any meaningful way.

The practitioners you meet are likely to be qualified in mental health practice and related specialities. You may be looking forward to widening your knowledge, but at the same time concerned that you will not understand your new colleagues because of the specialist nature of this work. If other students have told you about their ill-ease working in mental health, you may also wonder how you will be able to relate to the other staff (see Ch. 9).

These thoughts and self-knowledge will enable you to think of strategies to allay your anxieties and take some control over how you feel. Examples of some useful strategies for managing anxiety could be: travelling out to the unit so that you

Box 2.1 Going on a mental health placement

As a student, you are due to spend some time placed on a Day Unit for adults, such as new mothers, with mental illness. You probably have some ideas about what the experience will be like. In anticipation of any new placement (anticipatory reflection) it is useful to consider these ideas in some detail in order to clarify your thoughts and feelings, as they can influence your approach to the experience. Reflect on the following questions:

- How do you think people with mental illness will differ from people with physical illness?
- What other practitioners do you expect to be working with?
- How do you feel about working in this speciality?
- What experiences do you think underlie your expectations of this placement?
- With whom have you discussed your forthcoming placement?
- How do you think the conversations might have influenced your perceptions about this placement?

know exactly how to get there and how long it will take; arranging to introduce yourself to the midwife in charge before you begin your allocation; or reading up on the nature of mental health nursing. You might also find it reassuring to find out about the types of clients you will be meeting.

Model of reflection

As the development of effective communication skills for nursing and midwifery practice is the purpose of this text, Boud et al's (1985) model of reflection is chosen for the basis of this aspect of the book (Fig. 2.2). The model links well with the processes described by both Kolb (1975) and Benner (2001). It is also succinct and practice-focused, enabling the practitioner to reflect in a structured way, acknowledging all aspects of practice and their experiences, including those that may have been perceived as negative, as they can be transformed into positive action for the development of practice.

Another important aspect of how we think about our work, is the evidence-base that might have informed our understanding and/or decision-making. It can be helpful to identify on what principles we based our practice, such as the use of standard precautions to prevent infection and cross-infection in someone's home, and whether these principles were relevant and applicable in the situation you are reflecting upon. Sometimes you might find that, although you have applied the theory you knew, somehow it did not 'fit' your experience. This observation does not necessarily mean that there is no relevant research to help you understand your experience, and thus, perhaps, reinforces the spoken view that, 'what you learn in theory is irrelevant when you get out there and practise'! Your identification of gaps in your knowledge-base can help you to consider the evidence for practice that might be explained by another discipline such as sociology, psychology or management.

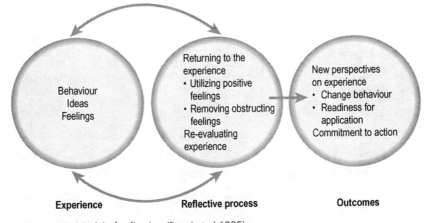

Figure 2.2 Model of reflection (Boud et al 1985).

Your experience of finding gaps in your knowledge and the evidence-base for practice can, in itself, help you to direct your reading and develop further your critical reflection and analytical skills in relation to the relevance of research. You might find particular studies and how they might be expanded and/or applied very useful to fill the gaps in your knowledge and application skills as well as identifying studies that perhaps were not appropriate because of the actual nature of the research, its ethics, process and/or conclusions and recommendations, thus enabling you to use research in a discriminating manner. This identification of areas where the evidence-base for practice is limited can indeed guide your own research projects (Taylor 2008).

On occasion, you or your colleagues may be involved in internal or external enquiries following episodes of practice that were found wanting. An essential premise of these enquiries is for **all** involved and others to learn from experience in order to avoid similar untoward events. Central to this process is the importance of relating professional practice to the standards set by the law, professional bodies, codes of practice and local protocols. Where protocols and practice are limited or inappropriate, they need to be reviewed and changed to incorporate new evidence. How we as practitioners then apply this new knowledge in our everyday work is our own responsibility, and it should be closely supported by continuing education and research.

Experience

This includes what we do, why we act as we do, what ideas we have and how we feel in any given situation in practice.

Reflective process

- **Returning to the experience** entails thinking back on the episode from practice and describing it. This description includes what we thought, felt and did at the time. By reviewing the experience in this structured way, we can become aware of observations, attitudes, feelings and thoughts that were preconscious or tacit, that is, not in the forefront of our awareness during the event.

- **Utilizing positive feelings**. By identifying the feelings that we had during the experience that enabled us, e.g. to respond sensitively and gave us the courage to stand up for our client, we can recognize and use these feelings to build on our future practice.

- **Removing obstructive feelings**. Any feelings such as disappointment, destructive self-criticism or a sense of not having done as well as we might have, can interfere with our capacity to review our experience with an open mind. These obstructive feelings may arise from unrealistic expectations of ourselves and others, or from being unwilling to accept that we are human and cannot practice perfectly all the time.

- **Re-evaluating the experience**. Once these feelings are acknowledged in the context of the positive feelings and of what actually happened in practice, the experience can be re-evaluated. Consequently, the reviewed perceptions of the episode that emerge offer us new insights into our experience.

Outcomes

New perspectives on experience are gained through the re-evaluation of the practice experience. These new perspectives allow us the opportunity to consider how to change our behaviour and so consider a variety of options for future practice in similar circumstances. Once we have clarified *what actions we can take* to develop our practice, it is important to be sure that we feel *ready* to apply our learning in practice. For reflection to have any effect on practice, we need to make a **commitment to action**; that is, we must be willing to change and develop our practice in the light of the new insights gained from the reflective process. It is through the linking of personal inner experience and the outer realities of our practice that we are able to re-frame our understanding of our work. These new insights can be used to review and apply the theory and evidence-base underpinning professional practice, with our personal experiences being a rich resource from which we can enhance our skills in the delivery of care.

As we reflect upon and transform our practice, so we are more able to demonstrate the evidence-base of our work, be accountable for our practice and autonomous within our professions. It is these essential characteristics that identify the power and authority of the competent professional practitioner.

During the reflective process, the re-enactment of what happens between the practitioner and the patient or client is frequently mirrored in the here-and-now processes between the supervisor and supervisee. This is known as the 'parallel process' and is enacted in supervision (Hawkins & Shohet 2006: 80–82). It mirrors in the here-and-now of the supervisory process, the professional practice processes-out-there and can be used to inform our reflections on practice. This complex phenomenon, if used effectively, can enlighten us about our professional development and practice – both in individual working relationships with clients, patients and colleagues, as well as within the organizations with which we work (Hawkins & Shohet 2006, Obholzer & Roberts 1994).

It is possible to relate the parallel processes of practitioner empowerment through knowledge and reflection to nurses' and midwives' commitment to the empowerment of those in their care, through effective communication, information-sharing and partnership in the process of care delivery. To this end, it is *crucial* that all practitioners have professional supervision in support of their development as reflective practitioners. This support can be in the form of one-to-one or group clinical supervision (Box 2.2).

Having answered these reflective questions, write a brief list of learning outcomes for tomorrow. Some examples of issues you might consider are below:

- The patients might have been more withdrawn than you anticipated. How can you go about making therapeutic relationships with them, as their needs are obviously different from patients you have cared for in the past? Who can help you develop these skills? What support do you think you will need?

- You might have found that you were reticent about asking staff about their specific roles and responsibilities. How do you intend to overcome this during

> ## Box 2.2 End of your first day
>
> You have now completed your first day in your new placement. Consider your expectations of the experience in relation to the realities of your first day.
>
> - You probably had some idea of how the patients would cope with their illnesses. How did your expectations match what you actually experienced when working with them?
> - When you started to make working relationships with the staff, what helped and what hindered this process? Were there specific anxieties that you anticipated that were not resolved? If so, what do you think the reasons for this might be?
> - How did you overcome any difficulties with new terminology?
> - What is the most significant piece of learning that you gained in your first day? How can you use this knowledge in placement in future?

your placement? What particular roles do you need to learn about? It may be helpful to think of strategies to engage staff in discussing their roles with you without it demanding excessive time. For example, when they are working with patients you might ask to observe alongside them, so that they can explain their roles to you while they work.

- You may think that it will be helpful to learn new terminology and what the actual diagnoses of the patients mean. Who can advise you on the best way to go about this? What textbooks are evident on the unit or have been recommended reading for this placement?

Your action plan for learning tomorrow and throughout the placement has thus been informed by your anticipatory reflections and can be developed from those at the end of your first day and subsequent days.

Reflective writing

An effective way to learn from practice and to make best use of your practice supervision is to keep a reflective journal. The aim of a reflective journal is to enable you to learn from your experiences throughout your professional life, by exploring them through regularly keeping a journal. This could be as stories, diagrams, maps, pictures or poetry. The reflective journal can be regarded as integral to the student's development, as learning from experience is fundamental to sound professional practice and lifelong learning. Practitioners are encouraged to keep reflective journals as supporting evidence for their continued professional development (Nursing and Midwifery Council 2008a).

To begin your journal, you may find it useful to choose an attractive book that feels special to you. Keep it solely for this purpose. In this, you record your thoughts, feelings, actions and experiences in your practice. Be frank with yourself and ask yourself what significance these particular experiences have for you and your development as a professional practitioner. Over the months, you are likely to see themes emerging which clarify your learning at particular stages in your progress as a nursing or midwifery student. Links may become apparent which would not have been evident had you not written thoughtfully, about your experiences in class and practice placements over a length of time.

Legal and ethical issues

In line with common practice, City University (2006) underlines legal and ethical issues surrounding professional practice, accountability and reflective journals. These issues are complex and have raised concerns in a number of professional arenas. It is therefore important to address the issues of confidentiality, disclosure and unethical practice in relation to the content of reflective journals.

On no account should details that could identify individuals, contexts and/ or situations relevant to cases about which you are writing *ever* be disclosed in your journal. The Nursing and Midwifery Council Code of Professional Conduct (Nursing and Midwifery Council 2008b) is very clear about this issue. You are accountable for knowing the limits of confidentiality in relation to your practice and the requirements of the laws in the countries in which you practice. It is important, too, that you take into account the implications of the Data Protection Act (1998) in anything you record.

The rules of **disclosure** in legal proceedings and courts of law can also apply to reflective journals. You should always be aware of this when writing your journal. It is therefore suggested that it is wise to reflect in writing or in other recording forms such as on a computer or if you use symbols, drawings or poetry, on issues that are unlikely to be the subject of case conferences, and/or legal proceedings.

Reflection on practice

The reflection on practice questions at the end of each chapter are not intended to be definitive, but are designed as a framework from which to review your experiences in practice and what you might consider in your reflections. They may also prove useful as a starting point for your reflective writing in your journal.

MENTORSHIP

It is best practice that all student nurses and midwives have a named mentor or, in situations where a one-to-one relationship is not possible, a co-mentor. Mentorship arrangements between students and qualified staff in their practice placements can be regarded as the first stage of supervision. By working alongside the qualified practitioners, the student learns the skills of nursing and midwifery practice. Relating practice to the learning outcomes for each placement is an integral part of providing structure for learning from experience and for developing the skills of reflection on experience.

The mentor's role is to support you in practice and enable you to learn from experience. In her seminal paper, Darling (1984) identified the 14 roles of the mentor. Among these are: a model for the student to admire and seek to emulate; an investor in the development of the student; a supporter who is empathetic to the needs of the student; a teacher-coach who shares expertise and skill; a problem-solver who helps the student explore problems and find solutions; and a challenger who encourages the student to think further and who questions views, attitudes and assumptions.

If you are to be helped to learn from practice, the core conditions necessary for any helping relationship, are important in the mentor–mentee relationship. These conditions are: involvement in the professional relationship between you and with the work; empathetic understanding; seeking order (from what might have felt like a chaotic or confusing experience); trust, respect, and a willingness to focus on the in-here phenomena, i.e. the capacity of the mentor to use the skills of immediacy (see Appendix 1) to address processes going on between you as a representation, or mirror, of what has happened out-there within an agreed working alliance with explicit focus and boundaries (Hazler & Barwick 2001). The relationship between you and your mentor may involve little choice about who will be working with whom, and it may need to be developed over a relatively short period of time. These factors might be problematic when the optimum practice climate for promoting reflection and effective mentorship – a 'welcoming, inquiring and reflective culture' (Sharp & Maddison 2008: 96) and thus for developing an effective working relationship – is not readily perceived by the student nor influenced by the mentor alone. In professional practice, however, you often have to make professional relationships with those in your care in a short space of time and within difficult situations. The skills used in the process of developing a relationship of trust and empathy in order to offer effective and responsive care to your clients and significant others, are those also used to develop the effective supporting relationship between mentor and mentee.

It is important, too, to recognize that the power differential between the student and the registered nurse or midwife also mirrors the power differential between the client and the professional practitioner. The student is the less experienced in the discipline and needs to rely on the qualified mentor to learn professional skills, just as patients and clients rely on the nurse's and midwife's superior knowledge and skills, to ensure they are cared for competently and to enable them to deal with their health issue.

THE SUPERVISION OF MIDWIVES

It is important to recognize the power differentials in supervision. Midwifery supervision is a statutory responsibility that provides a mechanism for support and guidance to every midwife practising in the UK (Nursing and Midwifery Council and the Local Supervising Authority (LSA) Midwifery Officers National

(UK) Forum 2008). The purpose of supervision is to protect women and their babies by actively promoting a safe standard of midwifery practice. The philosophy underpinning this statutory requirement is that supervision will be conducted in a manner which will foster openness and honesty, trust and reflection, and promote effective inter-professional communication. The supervisors are committed to supporting midwives in their professional development and therefore enhancing the professional role of the midwife, with the ultimate aim of providing care for mothers and babies that is safe and of a high standard (RCM 2008).

LEARNING CONTRACTS

In order to learn from practice, you are encouraged to develop a learning contract related to the learning outcomes for each placement. This is preferably negotiated with your mentor. Clear statements of what you want to learn, the actions necessary for you to gain the appropriate experience, what resources are available, the time span by which you will have met each learning outcome and the parameters for achievement and evaluation are important if your learning contract is to provide you with a framework for learning in practice. This contract will also provide you with a focus for thinking about your experiences, reflecting on what has happened, and considering how you can develop your practice further as a result of your learning through this process (Jarvis et al 2003, Ch. 10).

Your learning contract can support what you choose to review in your reflective journal. These strategies can provide you with rich resources from which to identify themes and issues in your professional development. They can enable you to plan your learning based on your experiences of what your strengths are and the areas you need to develop further. The skills you acquire from these processes will stand you in good stead throughout your professional career. The skills required to write a good learning contract are summarized in Box 2.3.

Clinical supervision

Butterworth & Faugier (1992) describe the process of support for the acquisition of nursing and midwifery skills and professional development. They outline the transition from mentorship for the pre-registration student to preceptorship for the newly qualified practitioner. The experienced practitioner would receive clinical supervision in a variety of different formats. Just as mentorship is the first stage of this process of reviewing practice and building on experience in order to learn professional skills in a supportive relationship with a registered colleague, qualified and experienced practitioners would seek clinical supervision that is at a different level compared with that received by the newly qualified person. The supervisor acts as a consultant (Hawkins & Shohet 2006) to the experienced practitioner through reflection within a formal and supportive relationship.

The purpose of reflection is the *development of practice* to the benefit of those in our care. It is therefore important to regard the supervision of practice in this

---

Box 2.3 | **Learning contracts**

The skills for writing learning contracts are:

Being specific

- about the overall aims and the component parts, i.e. the learning outcomes
- about resources needed to support learning, time frames and evaluation strategies
- about limits to practice, i.e. when skills should be practised with or without supervision.

Identifying learning outcomes and the processes of achieving them in the action plan.

Clarifying the outcomes and the processes of learning.

Being realistic

- in setting goals
- in time frames
- in the use of resources, including the involvement of colleagues
- in developing evaluation strategies.

Being honest about the process of achieving the learning outcomes. This is essential for:

- developing realistic action plans
- appropriate evaluation strategies
- obtaining appropriate support for your learning
- learning from reflection.

Negotiating skills in order to:

- develop a working partnership with your mentor/supervisor
- renegotiate the contract when unforeseen situations arise.

---

light. It differs from the emotional support we might seek after a demanding or distressing experience in either our personal or professional lives in that its focus is practice. It also differs from the oversight of managerial supervision where the practitioner's line manager gives the supervision and the relationship is one of supervisor–subordinate (Hawkins & Shohet 2006).

Butterworth & Faugier (1992) describe clinical supervision as an exchange between professionals in practice, enabling them to develop professional skills in order that practice is developed and sustained. The supervisory relationship is founded on trust and co-operation. To be optimally effective this relationship needs to be founded on the core conditions of effective helping relationships described by Rogers (1957) and discussed above and in Chapter 1. Proctor (1986) states that essential to the development of this relationship is the establishment of clear contracts of working between the supervisee and supervisor. These set boundaries to the relationship and are essential to the maintenance of psychological safety in the work (see Ch. 6). Proctor (1986: 27) identifies four aspects that are essential to this agreement:

1. The central focus is the working effectiveness of the student or worker.
2. The students or workers agree from the outset to recognize and accept responsibility for their own continuing development.
3. Any power or responsibility for assessment which the supervisor carries for the organization or profession with which both are connected is clearly spelt out and specified.
4. Both supervisor and student or worker recognize and agree to develop the skills appropriate to their respective roles.

This type of agreement makes clear the partnership inherent in supervision and mirrors the cooperative partnership practitioners develop with those in their care. Proctor (1986: 24) describes three processes inherent in supervision:

1. Formative – the development of skills through supervision;
2. Normative – the maintenance of standards of practice;
3. Restorative – the enabling of the supervisee to become 'refreshed' and become 'recreative'.

It is through these processes that supervisees reflect on their experience in practice, develop their skills and become increasingly self-aware. Therefore it is evident how the reflective process includes action, critical thought and the self, described above.

CONCLUSION

In order for you to develop as a practitioner and become increasingly skilled at relating theory to practice and to account for the evidence-base which has informed your decision-making, it is essential to reflect on your work. Integral to this process of professional development is the effective use of mentors, preceptors and clinical supervision. The use of clinical supervision in support of reflective practice is a fundamental component of nurses' and midwives' commitment to lifelong learning.

The sound supervisory relationship in many ways reflects the therapeutic relationship between practitioner and the client. It is through the use of reflection on practice, as well as on the development and maintenance of effective supervisory relationships, that practitioners are able to learn from experience and become reflective and creative practitioners, whose focus is the delivery of the best service possible to their clients and patients.

References

Benner, P., 2001. From Novice to Expert: Excellence and Power in Clinical Nursing Practice, commemorative edn. Addison Wesley Nursing Division, Menlo Park.

Boud, D., Keogh, R., Walker, D.R., 1985. Reflection: Turning Experience into Learning. Kogan Page, London.

Butterworth, T., Faugier, J., 1992. Clinical Supervision and Mentorship in Nursing. Chapman Hall, London.

City University, 2006. MSc in Interprofessional Practice Curriculum Documents. City University, London.

Darling, L.A., 1984. What do nurses want in a mentor? J. Nurs. Adm. 14 (10), 42–44.

Data Protection Act, 1998. HMSO, London.

Golman, D., 1998. Working with Emotional Intelligence. Bloomsbury, London.

Hawkins, P., Shohet, R., 2006. Supervision in the Helping Professions, 3rd edn. Open University Press, Buckingham.

Hazler, R.J., Barwick, N., 2001. The Therapeutic Environment. Open University Press, Buckingham.

Jarvis, P., Holford, J., Griffin, C., 2003. The Theory and Practice of Learning. 2nd edn. Kogan Page, London.

Johns, C., 2005. Expanding the gates of perception. In: Johns, C., Freshwater, D. (Eds.), Transforming Nursing Through Reflective Practice. Blackwell, Oxford.

Kolb, D.A., 1975. Experiential Learning. Prentice Hall, New Jersey.

Nurses', Midwives' and Health Visitors' Act, 1997. Online. Available at: www.opsi.gov.uk/ACTS/acts1997/ukpga_19970024_en_1 (accessed 19 July 2009).

Nursing and Midwifery Council and the Local Supervising Authority Midwifery Officers National (UK) Forum, 2008. Modern Supervision in Action a Practical Guide for Midwives. Online. Available at: www.nmc-uk.org/aDisplayDocument.aspx?documentID=3623 (accessed 19 July 2009).

Nursing and Midwifery Council, 2008a. The PREP Handbook (Revised). Nursing and Midwifery Council, London. Online. Available at: www.nmc-uk.org/aDisplayDocument.aspx? documentID=4340 (accessed 10 March 2009).

Nursing and Midwifery Council, 2008b. Code of Professional Conduct. Nursing and Midwifery Council, London. Online. Available at: www.nmc-uk.org/aArticle.aspx? ArticleID=3056 (accessed 13 March 2009).

Obholzer, A., Roberts, V.Z., 1994. The troublesome individual and the troubled institution. In: Obholzer, A., Roberts, V.Z. (Eds.), The Unconscious at Work: Individual and Organizational Stress in the Human Services. Routledge, London.

Proctor, B., 1986. Supervision: a co-operative exercise in accountability. In: Marken, M., Payne, M. (Eds.), Enabling and Ensuring: Supervision in Practice. National Youth Bureau, Leicester, pp. 21–34.

Rogers, C., 1957. The necessary and sufficient conditions of therapeutic personality change. J. Consult. Psychol. 21, 95–103.

Royal College of Midwives, 2008. Supervision of Midwives. RCM, London.

Schön, D.A., 1991. The Reflective Practitioner: How Professionals Think in Action. Basic Books, London.

Sharp, P., Maddison, C., 2008. An exploration of the student and mentor journey to reflective practice. In: Bulman, C., Schultz, S. (Eds.), Reflective Practice in Nursing. 4th edn. Blackwell, Oxford.

Sully, P., Wandrag, M., Riddell, J., 2008. The use of reflective practice on masters programmes in interprofessional practice with survivors of intentional and unintentional violence. Reflective Practice 9 (2), 135–144.

Taylor, B.J., 2008. Reflexivity: using reflection as an approach to research. In: Freshwater, D., Taylor, B.J., Sherwood, G. (Eds.), International Textbook of Reflective Practice in Nursing. Blackwell, Oxford.

van Manen, M., 1991. The Tact of Teaching, State of New York Press, New York.

Wilson, J.P., 2008. Reflecting-on-the-future: a chronological consideration of reflective practice. Reflective Practice 9 (2), 177–184.

Further reading

Bulman, C., Shultz, S., 2008. Reflective Practice in Nursing, 4th edn. Blackwell, Chichester.

Hughes, L., Pengelly, P., 1997. Staff Supervision in a Turbulent Environment: Managing Process and Task in Front-line Services. Jessica Kingsley, London.

Rolfe, G., Freshwater, D., Jasper, M., 2001. Critical Reflection for Nursing and the Helping Professions: a User's Guide. Palgrave, Basingstoke.

3

Ensuring respect and dignity

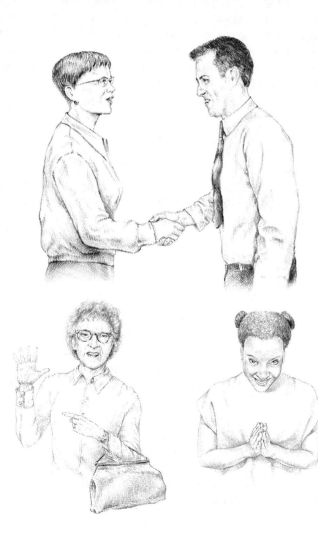

INTRODUCTION

Privacy and dignity are defined respectively as 'freedom from intrusion' and 'being worthy of respect' (Department of Health 2001: 204); both being identified 'as the softer aspects of care … which are nevertheless crucial to the quality of care patients experience' (Department of Health 2001: 10). In 2008, the Royal College of Nursing launched the 'Dignity at the heart of everything we do' campaign and emphasized that in order for people to feel comfortable and valued, it had to be an essential feature of the care and attention provided. In the absence of the three key elements of dignity: respect, compassion and sensitivity, people might '… lack confidence, be unable to make decisions for themselves and feel humiliated, embarrassed and ashamed' (Royal College of Nursing 2008: 1). Respect is identified as 'the foundation on which all helping interventions are built … a way of viewing oneself and others' (Egan 2007: 53). Egan (2007) considers that respect is a value that one holds and that dignity is a belief about how others should be treated. The norms that link these two aspects are outlined as ensuring that no harm is done, being competent and committed in one's work and being able to withhold judgement and by being person-centred.

It would be reasonable to assume that all humans welcome privacy and expect to be treated with dignity and respect. There are, however, many variables that will affect how these qualities are demonstrated and experienced. These variables include age, gender, status, culture, ethnicity and health status. When meeting patients, their relatives and other healthcare professionals for the first time, the practitioner needs to convey trust and a professional manner.

The scenarios in this chapter are presented to illustrate how practitioners might further develop their communication skills, in order to ensure respect and dignity while carrying out their work. The specific skills that are explored in this chapter include greeting adults and children, leave-taking skills and how to end relationships with colleagues.

GREETING SKILLS

When we meet people for the first time, the impression we make can be crucial for any continuing relationship with them. How we greet them is a significant part of this process. Berne (1975) explores the factors which influence what we say after we have said 'Hello'. While each person might have something to say, a number of considerations have to be taken into account in order for communication to be effective. The people with whom we come into contact might be anxious, frightened or angry. In the dementias, for example, memory and language are affected to different degrees, therefore as practitioners, making appropriate adjustments to our communication might help to address the person's concerns and facilitate an effective therapeutic relationship (Department of Health 2009). The dementias are '… acquired syndromes marked by chronic, global (not just memory and language problems) impairments of higher brain function occurring in alert patients which interfere with the ability to cope with daily living' (Nicholl 2006: 33).

Principles

When meeting patients/clients for the first time, it is important to introduce yourself and enquire about the identity of anyone else that might be with them. It is important to adjust the style of communication in accordance with the person or people with whom one is speaking. For example, if the person is deaf, practitioners should ensure that they stand at the side where the patient's hearing is best, face the patient and maintain good eye contact.

Social rules are learnt from within the context of one's upbringing and are integrated and activated at an unconscious level. It is therefore important for practitioners to increase their level of awareness with regard to meeting people from cultures different from their own in order to establish contact and reduce the risk of offence.

Forms of address vary across cultures, with some cultures placing higher regard on the use of titles than others. Individuals might feel offended if their full title is not used, since their title might denote status and possibly their occupation. It is important that practitioners also clarify how they would like to be addressed. Since there can be any number of different cultural groups in a large city, it would be unrealistic to be familiar with all of them. However, a lot can be learnt by observing the patient's preferred style of communication, the patient's use of eye contact and the extent to which they appear comfortable with your style of communication. The initial greeting can yield much information regarding the patient's level of understanding, degree of anxiety and support systems.

Greeting children and adults

You are a student nurse on a nursery placement and this morning you have just met an adult who has brought a child into the nursery.

Issues identified include:

- The importance of creating a good first impression
- How to help reassure individuals
- The need for familiarity concerning security procedures.

Specific principles

- When speaking with more than one person, it is imperative that communication is adjusted accordingly. For example, in this scenario the nurse might kneel down so as to be at the same level as the child.
- The parent might feel more at ease if they see that the child is settled and consider that you have the ability to care for their child. This latter aspect can be established if the nurse appears suitably dressed and presents an appropriate professional manner (see Ch. 6).

Preparation of self

- What is the correct procedure for receiving children into the nursery? Is there a book or form that needs to be completed before the child is left?
- What information do you have about the child/parent? What is their first language? Are they able to speak the formal language used in the nursery? If not, what resources are available that will assist your communication?
- Is the person accompanying the child their parent/guardian?
- What information do you need from the adult before they leave? For example, how has the child been over the last 24 hours? Has anything significant happened in the family that might affect the child's behaviour?
- What strategies does the nursery employ to reduce parents' anxiety during the early days of the child's stay in the nursery? For example, some nurseries send a fax of the child's drawing to reassure parents that their child has settled and is engaged in activities.
- Will you be the person spending time with the child during that day? If so, the parent might feel reassured to know this.

Environment

- The nursery environment can be one where the child feels secure and happy or where they are distressed and need longer to adjust.
- The parent might be unsure about leaving the child at the nursery, therefore it is important to present a warm, friendly and professional atmosphere.
- The environment also needs to take into account the cultural groups that the children represent, by providing facilities to ensure effective communication and development. Examples of this include the availability of toys that reflect the diversity of the children.

Putting the skills into practice

- Greet the adult both non-verbally, with a smile for example, and verbally by introducing yourself.
- Then greet the child using age-appropriate language; this might include involving any toys they might have with them in the conversation.
- Use short sentences if either the parent or the child speaks little English. If no English is spoken, an advocate/interpreter might be necessary.
- Find out how the child has been over the previous 24 hours.
- Posture, tone of voice and facial expression are very important, since there is a need to engage with both the adult and the child. This will also enable you to make an assessment of parenting style and the child's attachment style (Ainsworth et al 1978).

- Address any concerns that the parent might have, particularly if they are new to the nursery environment, and remind them of the activities that are available during the day.

- If the child is distressed, reassure the parent that this is normal and that the child will settle and that time will be spent with them until they do settle. Explain any measures that the nursery employs to put the child at ease since this might also reassure the adult.

- Confirm the arrangements for collecting the child and who will be collecting the child. If the adult who is collecting the child is not the parent, ensure that the procedure for this has been adhered to. For example this might include producing identification and confirming that the person has parental responsibility.

- Ensure that the procedure for leaving children at the nursery has been adhered to.

Reflection on practice

When meeting people of different ages, it is useful to reflect on your ability to adjust your communication appropriately and to assess the effectiveness of your communication style.

- How would you summarize your interaction with adults?
- How would you summarize your interaction with children?
- How would you reduce any anxieties that an adult might have about leaving a child?
- Similarly, how would you calm a child who is being left behind?
- If there are questions to which you do not know the answers, how will you get this information for future reference?
- How would you assess the relationship between an adult and a child? You might find it useful to discuss your thoughts with a qualified member of staff, to help you understand some of the principles of child development and child behaviour.

Orientating yourself to a new placement

In Chapter 2, you reflected on your expectations of a new placement as part of your preparation. Now think about how you would orient yourself as you start a new module and a new placement.

This scenario provides an opportunity to explore:

- The importance of preparation for new clinical placements
- How to create a good first impression
- How to generate motivation for new clinical experiences.

Specific principles

- An essential part of healthcare education and training is gaining experience in different clinical/practice placements. You might or might not be looking forward to working in some of the areas that your course has to offer; however, if you lack motivation while on a particular placement you might miss valuable learning opportunities. If you are finding it hard to be interested in the area you have been allocated to, aim to discuss this with a member of your support team, e.g. your mentor, link lecturer and/or personal tutor.

- A competent practitioner is one who works effectively as part of a team. Since the people that make up a team have a variety of personalities, it is the duty of each member to consider how they can best contribute to the effectiveness of the team (see Ch. 9).

- The ability to make and maintain relationships with other healthcare professionals is an essential skill. However, the breadth and depth of communication will vary according to the level of experience and familiarity with the individual and the environment.

- When meeting members of the team for the first time, it is important to introduce yourself and enquire about the identity of the others.

- Arriving on time is a crucial part of professional behaviour; therefore always allow plenty of time to travel to your placement.

Preparation of self

- Ensure that you have the correct start date, name and location of the placement area and the name of the person in charge.

- Contact the placement to establish your shift times and any other relevant geographic information.

- Familiarize yourself with the themes and foci of the module that accompanies this placement, as well as any assessments that need to be completed during this time.

- Acquaint yourself with the types of conditions/illnesses for which the patients/clients in that area are being seen/treated, and begin to consider any personal learning outcomes.

- Consider contacting your personal tutor or the link lecturer to help you prepare for the placement.

- Consult your reflective journal and comments from previous placements and devise a plan for addressing those areas that were identified and need to be addressed.

Environment

- The level of your previous clinical experience will determine the degree of familiarity you have with a ward or other placement environment.

- It is important to ascertain the exact location of those features common to most clinical environments, e.g. the treatment room, the sluice room and emergency equipment. There might also be equipment that is specific to the speciality with which you will need to become familiar.

Putting it into practice

- If you have not been able to visit the area before the start of your placement, arrive a few minutes early so that you can ascertain where to put your belongings and where the handover takes place.
- Introduce yourself and correct any errors in the pronunciation of your name.
- Limit your greeting of patients to non-verbal acknowledgements until you know more about them, unless there are obvious signs of distress, risk or emergency.
- Depending on the procedure in the clinical area, you might be introduced to other members of the team and patients/clients before, during or after the handover.
- Ensure that you clarify any pronunciations as they are given, e.g. if you are uncertain of the correct way to pronounce a person's name or a type of procedure.
- Use this opportunity as a preliminary assessment of both the social and psychological condition of the patients and the ward culture.
- You are likely to come across a number of new terms; make a note of those you do not understand and discuss them after the handover with your mentor or assessor or look them up later.
- Use this opportunity to undertake a preliminary assessment of both the social and psychological assessment of the patients/clients and the culture of the environment.
- In your introductions to patients/clients, inform them that you are a student; it might also be appropriate to inform them that it is your first day and a new area for you. Since patients have the right not to be cared for by students, your status as a student needs to be made explicit (Nursing and Midwifery Council 2002).
- It is important that you become orientated to the ward/area within the first few hours of arrival. This should include emergency procedures and telephone numbers, more detailed orientation would need to be completed by the first week.

Reflection on practice

During the early days of a new placement, it is important to reflect on the degree to which you are adjusting to the new environment and how this is contributing to your learning experience.

- By the end of the third day, to what extent do you feel familiar with the placement?

- What information do you still need and how are you going to get this information?
- What difficulties or challenges, if any, do you anticipate on this placement?
- When and where is the meeting with your mentor going to be held? (See Chapter 6 for more information about communicating with mentors.)
- Is there a link lecturer and when are they due to visit the placement next?
- What do you need to do to make the best of the learning opportunities available on the placement?
- When you think back to your first day on the placement, is there anything that you would have done or said differently?

Admitting a patient

A new patient has arrived on the ward and you have just greeted them and asked them to wait in the lounge area. The patient is from an ethnic background that is different from your own.

This scenario highlights a number of skills that can be used to facilitate an effective admission procedure. Admission to hospital causes patients varying degrees of anxiety. The practitioner who is admitting and orienting the patient has only one chance to make a good first impression. This process might present an additional challenge for both parties if they have different cultural norms.

Specific principles

In order to facilitate the development of an effective therapeutic relationship with individuals who are from an ethnic group that is different from your own, it is beneficial to become familiar with their preferred style of communicating. People from high-contact cultures, e.g. Southern Europeans and African-Caribbeans, might appreciate a handshake as a greeting more than those from low-contact cultures such as Chinese and East-Asian cultures (see Ch. 1). In recognition that there are a number of different cultural groups in a community, it is essential that attempts are made to ensure that the caring environment is equitable for all patients/clients with regard to actions taken to promote effective communication. An example of this would be the availability of cue cards reflecting the languages spoken by the patients who represent the community (see Ch. 7). While the practitioner might engage in information-gathering to increase effectiveness in communicating across cultures, it is important to remember that not all people coming from a specific culture observe the rites, rituals and customs that are identified as coming from that culture.

Most people admitted to a care environment are likely to experience a degree of anxiety. This is likely to be higher if they have been admitted as an emergency, since they have not had sufficient time to prepare themselves and mobilize their defences. The process of orienting a patient to the ward needs to take the mode of admission and the patient's condition into account. For example, is this an emergency admission or an elective one? Maslow's hierarchy of needs (Maslow 1954) provides a useful framework when considering the needs of the patient. For example, if the patient has a physiological need (they are hungry, need to go to the toilet or they are breathless), attention will need to be paid to this before continuing to discuss ward layout and procedures, thus meeting their safety and security needs. Maslow's (1954) hierarchy suggests that basic physical needs have to be satisfied before moving to higher-order needs.

The initial greeting can yield much information regarding the patient's level of understanding, degree of anxiety and their support systems. For example, is the patient accompanied by anyone? Is their body language congruent with their responses, e.g. do they say they are fine but appear tense and worried?

Preparation of self

- What information do you have about the patient?
- What is the first language of the patient/client? What dialect do they speak? You might need to arrange for an interpreter or have cue cards available that reflect the patient's language (see Ch. 7).
- What is the patient's name, age and reason for admission?
- Is the patient's bed area appropriately prepared? For example, is the area clean and is the bed ready if the patient wishes or needs to lie down? Is there water, if appropriate? Does any equipment need to be available for the patient?
- Will you be the person admitting the patient? If so, ensure that you have the necessary documentation with you.
- If you will not be the person carrying out the admission procedure, you will need to explain this to the patient. This would be an ideal learning opportunity for you to observe your mentor/assessor or to be observed by your mentor/assessor while carrying out this procedure.

Environment

- The ward environment is one with which you need to become increasingly familiar and comfortable. This familiarity includes the acceptance of the noises, sights, smells and routines that are a part of the work environment, and recognition of any deviations from the norm.
- There also needs to be an awareness of how these features of a ward might affect someone who is not as familiar with them as you are.
- The ward environment needs to provide a secure (both physically and psychologically) space where patients can trust that they will be cared for.
- Each member of the team, whether based on the ward or not, e.g. a physiotherapist, contributes to the ward environment.
- Box 3.1 summarizes the process for orienting a patient to the ward.

> ### Box 3.1   Checklist for the orientation of a patient to a ward
>
> - Personal introductions including student status. It would also be appropriate to identify the various people and their uniforms
> - Introduction to the layout of the ward
> - Identification of their bed space and surrounding areas
> - Introduction to the nearest patient/client as appropriate
> - Location of the bathrooms, toilets, dayroom. Colours and symbols that are used to highlight important areas are particularly useful if the patient/client has a dementia/or speaks a different language
> - Routines regarding the availability of refreshments, reading materials (TV and radio), making and receiving telephone calls and mealtimes
> - General ward routines
> - Guidance regarding what to do if they want to leave that ward, i.e. to go to the shop, chapel, etc.
> - Procedure for the safe storage of property and valuables
> - The availability of resources, such as an interpreter, religious/spiritual representatives
> - The availability of an aspect of care the patient/client might be concerned about, e.g. pain control.

Putting the skills into practice

- Introduce yourself and clarify with the patient how they would like to be addressed.
- The order in which you orient the patient will need to take into account the condition of the patient. The process might need to be conducted over the course of the day.
- Since orientation to the ward is part of the admissions procedure, ideally the practitioner who does this should be the one who conducts the initial patient assessment as well as completing relevant documentation.
- This would provide both you and the patient/client with a degree of continuity. It might be more practicable, however, if the process of orientation and admission is shared between you and your mentor/assessor.
- As locations are pointed out to the patient and routines explained, note how the patient is responding to the information, both verbally and non-verbally. Use these moments to offer clarification and reassurance.
- When asking questions, ensure that you do not use multiple questions since this can lead to confusion, as you will not be sure which question the individual is answering (see Ch. 5).

- The development of a therapeutic relationship will be dependent on the patient's/client's experience of feeling cared for. As a practitioner you can enhance the quality of the relationship by demonstrating empathic understanding and acceptance. For example, you might say: *'The bed probably isn't what you're used to, but we'll try and make you as comfortable as possible.'*

- The aim of demonstrating the core conditions of empathic understanding, genuineness and acceptance is to help reduce the patient's/client's experience of any physical and/or psychological pain they might be experiencing. This can be achieved by remaining calm, demonstrating the ability to act appropriately and engaging in effective problem-solving. For example, by suggesting a change in position to relieve any pain the patient/client might have.

- If the patient is anxious or in pain, touch might be a useful intervention. In this case it might also be appropriate to use more closed rather than open questions, e.g. *'Would it help if I sat with you for a short while?'* or *'Is that better?'*

- If relatives are present and they have been instrumental in assisting you with communicating with the patient/client, consider asking them to write down common phrases that can aid communication when an interpreter or relative is not available.

- It would also be valuable if any specific preferences/practices that the client/patient might have/needs to observe are explored. For example, these might relate to diet, hygiene needs or worship. However, when involving relatives in interpreting, the patient's confidentiality needs to be considered and protected.

- It is not uncommon that people who do not have English as a first language might be able to speak some English but feel less comfortable communicating in English. The practitioner could facilitate the client's confidence by encouraging them and giving them feedback.

- If communicating via an interpreter or translator, it is important to maintain eye contact with the patient/client while speaking with the interpreter or translator. This might feel awkward but it will ensure you remain in connection with the patient (see Ch. 7).

- It is important to establish who should be contacted if there is a change in the patient's/client's condition.

Reflection on practice

- Having admitted a patient/client, it is important to reflect on this process, not only because something might have been forgotten, but also to evaluate your effectiveness during this first meeting.

- What have you learnt from your initial meeting with this patient/client and, if accompanied, from their relative/s?

- What is the patient's/client's level of understanding of their environment and the reason for their admission?

- Were there any communication difficulties? If so, how do you think these can be addressed during the patient's/client's stay?

- How would you sum up the relationship between the patient/client and their relative? This information might give you some insight into the patient's/client's close relationships, their support system and their degree of dependence or independence, both physical and psychological.
- Did the patient/client and/or relative express any concerns that you were not able to address? If so, what were they and what do you need to do about this?
- How would you rate the relationship between you and the patient/client and vice versa?
- Has all the necessary information been documented?
- Looking back at your first meeting with a patient/client, was there anything that you could have done or said differently?
- Which elements of undertaking a cultural assessment do you need to familiarize yourself with?

Use of terminology in obstetric emergencies

You are caring for a woman called Patricia, while she is in labour. When you examine her you find she has a prolapsed cord. You know that this means her baby is at extreme risk and could die unless you intervene immediately. You also know that you need to ask her to adopt what is often described as asking the woman to 'get on all fours with her bottom in the air' position, in order to take the pressure off her baby's umbilical cord. You explain the findings of your examination and give her instructions about the position she needs to adopt to take the pressure off the umbilical cord.

Some issues raised by this scenario:

- This situation is an obstetric emergency. It is in these circumstances that communication is most likely to be delivered in short specific directives to the woman.
- While this is a very important instruction, the midwife needs to be very sensitive as to how it might be received and perceived.
- The woman is likely to be very anxious because of the risk to her baby and herself. She might be aware also of a sense of increased powerlessness and vulnerability, which might be reminiscent of past experiences of abuse or indeed of the circumstances of her baby's conception.
- The instruction to 'get on all fours' could well remind her emotionally and/or cognitively of previous occasions when she was in a humiliating and/or non-consensual sexual situation and one where she thought her life might be at risk, i.e. situations which might be reminiscent of past sexual abuse.

- If she reacts in what might be considered as an 'unco-operative manner', i.e. freezes or refuses to adopt the position, it might indicate distress. Her response might not be related to the here-and-now but is an unconscious defence for self protection as a result of the negative transference with the midwife who could be perceived in the same light as the past abuser. The gender of the midwife might well affect the response. For further discussion on the impact of the transference on the therapeutic relationship, see Chapter 1.

Environment

- There is likely to be an increase in the number of people and the amount of equipment in the room. Any newcomers should introduce themselves or be announced by the midwife and their presence explained.
- Noise can be very anxiety provoking. It is important to keep this to a minimum to ensure the environment conveys a sense of respect for the woman and what is happening to her and her baby.
- The temperature of the room needs to be appropriate and comfortable for the woman and suitable for her baby.

Preparation of self

- Although this type of situation cannot be anticipated in relation to a specific woman's labour, it is important for the midwife to reflect upon how they might feel, what they should do and how they intend to respond when faced with this type of obstetric emergency. Anticipatory reflection (Sully et al 2008) enables practitioners to plan ahead for foreseen and unforeseen events.
- Acknowledgement of one's feelings such as fear, excitement, anticipation allows for the development of effective coping strategies that will not interfere with offering optimum care in emergencies.

Putting it into practice

- It is important to establish eye contact with the woman when you give her the instruction to change her position.
- Language that you could use instead of the term, 'Please get on all fours' could be *'Please kneel and then lean forward on to your forearms so your shoulders are lower than your hips.'*
- It might be appropriate to follow-up this instruction with a cue card or drawing of the position the woman needs to adopt (see Appendix 3).
- It is important to respond sensitively to any manifestations of distress or confusion throughout this process. Using a well-modulated and gentle voice, alongside a calm and efficient approach can induce confidence in the woman.
- Wherever possible, it is important to offer the woman choices when the situation is being managed, e.g. *'Would you like a blanket to keep you warm?'*

- It is essential for the midwife to observe the woman's non-verbal behaviour in relation to where other people are positioned in the room. Where people are not involved in her actual physical care, it is important to ensure that they position themselves where the woman feels at ease.

Reflection on practice

- Following an emergency it is likely that you will feel a mixture of emotions about how you delivered care, the outcome of the situation and the effects it has had on you and your colleagues. Think about a situation when you were involved in delivering care during an emergency. How did you feel when you became aware that the situation was life-threatening? How did this influence the ways in which you reacted?
- How did you maintain the client's dignity and demonstrate respect for them?
- What helped and/or hindered your ability to maintain the client's dignity?
- It is likely that you had learnt about emergency care prior to actually dealing with the situation. Were there any emotional and/or practice aspects that you had not anticipated?
- What have you learnt about yourself and your ability to manage yourself in emergencies? How will this awareness influence your future practice?

Communicating with an older adult with dementia

Mrs James (Sarah) is an 84-year-old woman who has been on the ward for 3 days. Mrs James lives at home with her husband, but was admitted because she sustained an injury to her leg, having fallen while wandering around the house late one night. Mrs James has late stage Alzheimer's disease and it is becoming increasingly difficult for her husband (Fred), who has poor eyesight, to manage things at home. They have two children who live a distance away, a son (Robert) and daughter (Mary), who both visit weekly.

You are on a late shift and discover that Mrs James is banging and shouting at a door and looking generally distressed. You approach her.

Specific principles

- The older patient might have some communication difficulties, which may range from a hearing or sight impairment, to aphasia or dysarthria. The latter might have resulted from a stroke or other neurological disorder.
- In the dementias, memory impairment and preservation (the repetition of previous information that is not relevant to the current context), is a common feature, therefore it is important to be patient and clear in your

communication and to facilitate the patient to engage in conversation (Bayles & Tomoeda 2007).

- Ensure that any aids the patient might need to facilitate effective communication are available, e.g. dentures that fit correctly, a hearing aid with a functioning battery.
- Older people might have difficulty with long sentences; therefore consider how you structure your sentence to ensure the main points are identified in a concise manner. It might be necessary to repeat the focus of the conversation.
- Communication will be more effective if you use normal intonation, appropriate timing and emphasis on relevant words. With regards to pace, it might be appropriate to speak at a slightly slower pace with pauses which would enable the listener to process the information. However, if the pace is too slow, the patient might find it difficult to remember the earlier part of the conversation.
- While a slower pace might be used, it is important not to sound patronising and to ensure that a childlike tone or language is avoided.
- During the course of the day (e.g. following a wandering incident), it might be necessary to re-orientate the patient about where they are and why they are there.
- While carrying out care it might also be appropriate to involve any mementoes Mrs James might have brought from home. In your conversations with her, you can use these mementoes as a means of helping her to remember her past in a positive way.
- Since it might be difficult for a person with a dementia to generate possible responses to open questions, it is more effective to use open focused questions which will encourage choices to be made (see Chapter 5). For example:

'What would you like to wear today?' would be better as: 'Which dress would you like to wear today, the pink one or the yellow one?'

- Effective communication also needs to take place in a context: so in the above conversation if the nurse is helping the patient with hygiene needs and has both dresses in her hands, this helps the patient to grasp the information.
- Care needs to be taken, however, to ensure that the patient is not required to concentrate on more than one thing at a time, e.g. asking them about their choice of clothes, while also asking them to carry out an activity.
- If it appears that the person has not understood what has been said, this will need to be restated in a different way.
- If the person has difficulty remembering events (episodic memory), it can be helpful to use proper nouns rather than pronouns. For example, rather than:

'Robert and Mary went to see Fred yesterday and the district nurse was there. They wanted to make sure everything was alright and she said he was fine.'

The following would be easier for the person to understand:

'Robert and Mary went to see Fred yesterday and the district nurse was there. Robert and Mary wanted to make sure everything was alright and the nurse said Fred was fine.'

- As with all effective exploratory communication, engaging the five senses is very useful, e.g. *'Does this feel soft?'*, *'Is the radio too loud for you?'*, *'Does this smell like tea or coffee?'*
- It might also be difficult for the patient if a number of people are speaking at once, e.g. during an interdisciplinary team meeting.
- While use of humour can be appropriate, the person with a dementia might not be able to interpret the meaning and therefore there might be a risk of being disrespectful towards the individual.
- It is important to check the side-effects of any medication that Mrs James might be taking, since these might contribute to her feelings and behaviour.

Preparation of self

- What is your aim as you approach Mrs James?
- What is her aim?
- How do the two conflict?
- How are you going to address this? What words might you use?

Environment

- Be alert to the level of noise that might be in the nearby area, since this can cause the patient to become agitated.
- Are there any potential risks in the vicinity?
- The level of lighting needs to be reduced when helping the patient settle for bed.

Putting it into practice

- Approach Mrs James in a calm, unhurried manner and consider your body language, since you do not want to startle her.
- Remind Mrs James of your name and your role.
- It might be appropriate to touch her arm and then ask her if you can take her hand, you might also indicate that this is what you want to do.
- Link the information that is being communicated with information that is already known, this will involve some degree of repetition, e.g. *'Mrs James remember you are in hospital? Are you looking for your bed or do you need to go to the toilet?'*
- If you do not understand her response, you can use closed questions and/or gestures to try and capture/guess what she is trying to say.
- It would also be appropriate to acknowledge her feelings and validate them, e.g. *'I can see you're very upset, are you in pain?'* or *'Were you looking for the way to your home?'*
- In order to help Mrs James re-orientate to the time and location, you might give her some information. This should be in manageable chunks and you

will need to check her understanding. For example: *'You're on the ward and it's night time. I can help you get ready for bed. Your bed is over there, shall we go now?'*

- At an appropriate point, it would be important to check that Mrs James has not sustained any injuries during this episode.

Reflection on practice

- When working with a patient who has a dementia, how have you been able to involve them in their care and find out what they want?
- How have you encouraged a patient with dementia to engage in conversation with staff, other members of the team, their relatives?
- Are there areas related to cognitive impairment and neurological disorders that might help you further understand a patient's communication difficulties?

LEAVE-TAKING SKILLS

The skills of taking our leave are as important as greeting skills in all professional relationships. The non-verbal gestures and terms of address we choose will, of course, be dictated by the nature of the relationships we have with the people involved and each unique circumstance. This might be formal or informal, depending on the nature and significance of the relationship. Achieving closure and ending professional relationships with groups, e.g. at the end of your education programme, is addressed in Chapter 9.

Specific principles

- When leave-taking, you need to adjust your style of language and non-verbal cues to take into account the age, gender and culture of the people involved, as well as the nature of your relationships with them.
- Using the core conditions of effective therapeutic relationships addressed in Chapter 1, it is possible to disagree on issues without losing respect for the other people involved. Leave-taking in these circumstances might be difficult if tempers are running high; however it is possible to focus on what has been achieved, such as an agreement to disagree.
- When taking our leave, it is important to acknowledge something positive that has been gained from the experience of working with the others involved. This is especially important when the relationships have not run smoothly.
- This skill of focusing on the positive when ending professional relationships, allows for the possibility of those involved to remember the encounter in a positive way. This is especially important when patients and clients have lived through frightening and painful experiences that you have shared with them.

- Leave-taking can raise paradoxical feelings of loss as well as relief that a difficult time has come to an end, or pleasure at looking forward to a new phase in life such as when a new mother goes home with her partner and their baby.

Saying goodbye

You are due to finish your shift and have been nursing a 45-year-old patient, Mr Alphonso, for the last 2 weeks. He is due for open-heart surgery in the morning. He will be admitted to the Intensive Care Unit when he leaves theatre. You are aware that he is understandably anxious about the operation. You are also unlikely to be nursing him again because when he returns to the ward you will have moved to a new practice placement.

Some issues raised by this scenario:

- Mr Alphonso is facing major surgery, which everyone hopes will greatly improve his quality of life; however it also carries a significant risk to his health. You know he is anxious about this and the possibility that he could die.
- The symbolism of your not seeing him again could raise for him associations between parting and death.
- There is fear of the unknown, e.g. in Mr Alphonso's feelings about being in intensive care and away from being nursed in a familiar environment by a familiar nurse.
- You need to acknowledge your feelings about saying goodbye to a patient at a time when he is vulnerable and facing a stressful life event.
- There are parallel processes of your moving on to a new and stressful but probably positive experience as you progress through your programme, and Mr Alphonso facing a new and stressful experience.

Preparation of self

- Think about your feelings in relation to this situation. You might well have been in similar situations before with patients and clients.
- How do you feel about saying goodbye to Mr Alphonso, especially bearing in mind that you have supported him in preparation for this surgery?
- What do you think you offered him that he seems to have especially valued when having been nursed by you?
- What have you gained from nursing him? Perhaps you have enjoyed his sense of humour or he has told you interesting things about his family, background and culture.

- What do you think he is likely to miss about being away from the ward? How will this knowledge influence what you will say to him when you take your leave?
- What physical gestures will you consider using, e.g. shaking hands, sitting beside his bed?

Environment

- Consider the best place and time in which to take your leave of Mr Alphonso.
- Where are you going to say goodbye? Will you talk to him by his bed or take him into an interview room if the ward has one?
- Who can overhear you? Does it matter if the conversation is not private? These considerations will be affected by the strength of the bond you have with Mr Alphonso and how much he has shared his experiences with you.
- It is best practice to ensure as much privacy as possible.

Putting the skills into practice

Once you have decided when and where you are going to take your leave, you need to decide on how to perform the skill.

- Make time for the ending.
- Decide what you are going to say and how you are going to say it.
- What physical gestures will you feel comfortable using? Decide whether you will sit down or stand.
- Be empathetic to how Mr Alphonso might be feeling about his situation and about saying goodbye to you. Warmth and politeness when saying goodbye help to avoid the implication of rejection.
- Say goodbye, using clear language that means the encounter is ending. Avoid euphemisms such as 'see you later' when this is unlikely to happen.
- Sometimes patients and clients keep in touch with the ward by letter or telephone (this might be necessary for follow-up treatment or support). However, it is important to avoid encouraging inappropriate dependence.
- If the patient is being referred elsewhere, clarify the arrangements with him before you say goodbye.
- Include any family or friends of the patient who are present, especially if you have had significant dealings with them.
- Acknowledge the significance of the relationship to you, by valuing expressed feelings and stating your own, e.g. *'It has been a privilege to ...'*
- Give space by leaving time and remaining quiet for Mr Alphonso to give you feedback on his experiences of being cared for by you.

- When actually parting, be culturally sensitive in what physical gestures you use, e.g. bowing or waving.
- Where possible, if others are leaving, escort them to the door and open it. If you are leaving someone's home, it is important to allow them to open their own door and see you out.

Reflection on practice

- How successful were you in your preparation for taking your leave?
- What aspects of the environment where you took your leave were appropriate? Where the environment was not ideal, what did you do to ensure that it was possible for your leave-taking to be the focus of the interaction between you and Mr Alphonso and be managed respectfully?
- How did you feel before, during and after saying goodbye to Mr Alphonso? What do you think the reasons were for this?
- How do you think these feelings might have influenced your non-verbal cues, the language you used and how he experienced the process?
- In what ways did cultural awareness influence what you said and did? For example, did you shake his hand?
- What have you learned from this experience? How will you develop your practice as a consequence of this reflection?

Ending relationships with colleagues

For the last 4 weeks you have worked in the community with the district nurses or midwives. During this placement you have worked with all the nurses or midwives in the team, but you have spent most of the time with the Team Leader. Today is your last day in this placement.

Some issues raised by this scenario:
- The influence that experience and status have on your relationships with team members and their attitudes towards teaching students.
- Which nurse or midwife completes the practice-based assessment for your placement?
- The length of time in the placement as well as the amount of time worked with particular individuals.
- The levels of formality and informality in the community compared with hospital placements, e.g. in some Primary Care Trusts nurses and midwives do not wear uniforms when caring for patients or clients in their homes.
- The importance of acknowledging what they have offered and what you have gained from working with them.

Preparation of self

- Think about how you are feeling at the prospect of leaving this placement and the colleagues with whom you have worked. Your feelings are likely to be mixed: are you sorry or relieved to be going?
- How did you experience working in the community? What was particularly significant learning for you?
- If you found it more difficult to build rapport with some colleagues, acknowledge what you have learnt from them as a way of ending the relationship positively.
- How will you integrate these thoughts and feelings into what you will say to your colleagues?

Environment

- In deciding how you are going to take leave of your colleagues, you need to consider the best place and time in which to do it.
- Decide if you intend to speak to all the members of the district nursing or midwifery team together. If this is not possible, whom will you contact?
- If you are saying goodbye over the telephone, who can overhear you? Does it matter if the conversation is not private? For example, you might want to acknowledge a shared confidence.

Putting the skills into practice

Once you have decided when and where you are going to take your leave, you need to decide on how to perform the skill.

- Make time for the ending.
- Decide what you are going to say and how you are going to say it.
- Decide on your non-verbal gestures.
- Be empathetic to how the other people involved might be feeling about their situations and about saying goodbye to you. Warmth and politeness when saying goodbye help to avoid the implication of rejection.
- Say goodbye, using clear language that means the encounter is ending. Avoid euphemisms such as 'see you later' when this is unlikely to happen.
- Acknowledge the significance of the relationships to you, by valuing expressed feelings and stating your own, e.g. *'I have really enjoyed working with all of you in the community. I have learnt how exciting it is to work with a committed and integrated team. I'll miss you all.'*
- Give space for the team members to give you feedback about their experiences of working with you as a student.
- When actually parting, be culturally sensitive in what physical gestures you use with each team member, for example, by shaking hands or waving.

- If others are leaving you and it is your space, escort them to the door and open it. If you are leaving your colleagues' office, it is important to allow them to open the door and see you out, whenever possible. Who sees who to the door is an unspoken norm in different situations. It is important to be aware of the customs in each of your placements.

Reflection on practice

- How successful were you in your preparation for taking your leave?
- What aspects of the environment where you took your leave were appropriate?
- Where the environment was not ideal, what did you do to ensure that it was possible for your leave-taking to be the focus of the interaction and managed respectfully?
- How did you feel before, during and after the parting?
- How do you think these feelings might have influenced your non-verbal cues, your tone of voice and the language you used?
- How do you think your colleagues experienced the process? What happened for you to come to these conclusions?
- In what ways did cultural awareness influence what you said and did?
- How will you develop your practice as a consequence of this reflection?

References

Ainsworth, M., Blehar, M., Waters, E., Wall, S., 1978. Patterns of Attachment: A Psychological Study of the Strange Situation. New Jersey, Erlbaum.

Bayles, K., Tomoeda, C., 2007. Cognitive-communication Disorders of Dementia. Plural, Oxford.

Berne, E., 1975. What Do You Say After You Say Hello? Corgi, London.

Department of Health, 2009. Living Well with Dementia: A National Strategy. Department of Health, London.

Department of Health, 2001. The Essence of Care. Department of Health, London.

Egan, G., 2007. The Skilled Helper: A Problem-management and Opportunity-development Approach to Helping. Brooks/Cole, Pacific Grove.

Maslow, A., 1954. Motivation and Personality. Harper & Row, New York.

Nicholl, C., 2005. Mental health in older age. In: Bryan, K., Maxim, J. (Eds.), Communication Disability in the Dementias. Wiley Blackwell, Chichester.

Nursing and Midwifery Council, 2002. An NMC Guide for Students of Nursing and Midwifery. Nursing and Midwifery Council, London.

Royal College of Nursing, 2008. Campaign on Dignity (continuing), Online. Available at: www.rcn.org.uk/newsevents/campaigns/dignity (accessed 7 July 2009).

Sully, P., Wandrag, M., Riddell, J., 2008. The use of reflective practice on masters programmes in interprofessional practice with survivors of intentional and unintentional violence. Reflective Practice 9 (2), May 2008, 135–144.

Further reading

Bryan, K., Maxim, J., (Eds.), 2005. Communication Disability in the Dementias. Wiley Blackwell, Chichester.

Dunhill, A., Elliott, B., Shaw, A., (Eds.), 2009. Effective Communication with Children and Young People, their Families and Carers. Learning Matters, Exeter.

Milner, P., Carolin, B., 1999. Time to Listen to Children: Personal and Professional Communication. Routledge, London.

Nelson-Jones, R., 2006. Human Relationship Skills, 4th edn. Routledge, London.

Petrie, P., 1997. Communicating with Children and Adults: Interpersonal Skills for Early Years and Playwork. Edward Arnold, London.

Richardson, J., Burnard, P., 1994. Talking with children: some basic counselling skills. Prof. Care Mother Child 4, 111–114.

Rogers, C., 1957. The necessary and sufficient conditions of therapeutic personality change. J. Consult. Psychol. 21, 95–103.

Socha, T., Stamp, G., 2009. Parents and Children Communicating with Society. Routledge, London.

Vangelisti, A., 2003. Handbook of Family Communication. Routledge, London.

4

Empathy and comfort skills

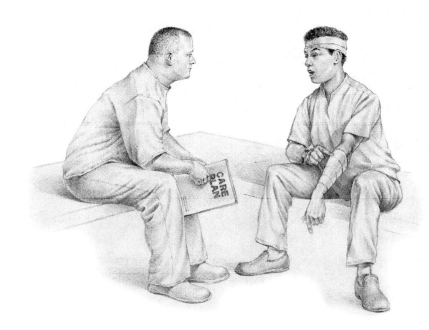

INTRODUCTION

Compassion is at the heart of nursing and midwifery practice (Royal College of Nursing 2008). In order to communicate this value, practitioners need to be responsive to the social, psychological, emotional and spiritual as well as physical needs of those in their care. The practitioner–client relationship is central to the delivery of care. By the sensitive use of verbal and non-verbal skills, we can offer the core conditions of all therapeutic relationships to patients and clients – warmth and respect, empathetic understanding, openness and genuineness (Rogers 1957) (see also Ch. 1). For these reasons, we need to develop our emotional intelligence so that we are self-aware, aware of the needs of those in our care, and aware of the circumstances in which we are involved. Golman (1998: 317) describes emotional intelligence as, 'the capacity for recognizing our own feelings and those of others, for motivating ourselves, and managing emotions well in ourselves and in our relationships'.

THE PRACTITIONER–CLIENT RELATIONSHIP

Sundeen et al (1998) identify the components of the nurse–client relationship as:

- Valuing: recognizing one's own values and respecting others' values
- Trust: a sense that others are able to assist in a time of distress
- Empathy: the capacity to be with a client and perceive accurately her or his feelings, experience and meaning
- Caring or love: unconditional acceptance of the other as she or he is
- Hope: the expectation of good in the future while recognizing the uncertainty of the future
- Autonomy and mutuality: the ability to be self-determining as well as sharing with others.

When we respond compassionately to those in our care we recognize their need for comfort, and we are able to do so because we have an empathetic understanding of their needs.

Empathy

Empathy is often defined as putting yourself in someone else's shoes. In this position, however, you ensure that the other person will go barefoot! This means they are disadvantaged and their autonomy could be compromised by our taking over their situation, even although we are trying to be compassionate and caring. Empathy is therefore better described as being alongside those in our care in order to be sensitive to their 'feelings', 'experience' and 'meanings' (Sundeen et al 1998: Ch. 5). Benner (2001: 70) describes this as 'The nurse is *with* the patient without fusing her [sic] own boundaries, selfhood, or integrity. Nurses are not endangered by the patient's perceptions or behavior' (Benner 2001: 70, original italics).

As empathy requires us to be self-aware and self-regulating, it is important that when we reflect-in and on-action we use our own emotions to help, rather than hinder, our abilities to address effectively the situations in which we are currently involved (see Ch. 2). As a result of unconscious psychological processes in people's motivation and relationships, particularly the transference relationship (i.e. unconscious responses to others as if they were significant people from our past), lack of awareness can prompt inappropriate responses to others, to the feelings others and the situations evoke in us (see Ch. 1). Self-awareness and self-regulation can enable us to learn from experience and develop our personal and professional skills, in order to be empathetic and offer comfort more sensitively.

Arguably, these principles apply in *all* healthcare, in that we work with people in need, they come to us when they are vulnerable – physically and/or emotionally – and they ask for our professional involvement at a time of significance to them.

Comfort

Comfort means: 'Relief or support in mental distress or affliction; consolation, solace, soothing' (*Oxford English Dictionary* 1989 Online). Christensen (1993: 116–117) describes part of the work of the nurse as 'attending', that is, being present, ministering, listening, comforting; she also describes 'enabling' those in our care as integral to giving comfort. In attending, we can offer comfort by using our empathy to inform our communication in nursing and midwifery practice. We soothe and console by our informed and sensitive use of verbal and non-verbal skills.

The scenarios in this chapter are presented to illustrate how practitioners might develop their communication skills further, in order to give empathy and comfort while carrying out their work. The specific skills that are explored here include: paraphrasing skills; the appropriate use of touch; awareness of cultural differences in the expression of distress; ensuring privacy and dignity; and providing emotional support when those we care for are experiencing intense feelings such as fear, anger and pain.

PRINCIPLES

In order to demonstrate empathy and to offer comfort, we need to consider a number of principles. When our words are congruent with our non-verbal and paralinguistic communication, others are more likely to experience us as genuine and open because we are less likely to be giving mixed messages. **The skills addressed below should always be used in a relationship of respect and concern.** If they are used as 'clever tricks' to pretend that we are listening in order to cover up our unwillingness to help with someone's problems, we are likely to be unsuccessful at offering empathy and comfort and, at worst, could cause offence or hurt.

Self-awareness

People in distress or need can be very dependent on those who care for them. The practitioner–client relationship is, by its very nature, intimate (Kadner 1994). Nurses and midwives are allowed into emotional, physical and spiritual places where few others, except perhaps the most important people in clients' lives, are welcome. In order to avoid exploiting, however unintentionally, the power this gives us, we need to be very aware of the privilege we are granted by being there with people at significant times in their lives. It is therefore essential that we are prepared, throughout our professional lives, to develop our self-awareness, reflect on our work and maintain the humility that enables us to learn from practice.

The core conditions of helping (warmth and acceptance, empathy, openness and genuineness) are fundamental to all compassionate and trusting professional relationships. The capacity to 'be with' (Benner 2001: 50) those in our care, demands that we listen attentively to both their words and their non-verbal cues, e.g. choice of words, posture or physical signs, or paralinguistic changes such as tone of voice.

Demonstrating this ability takes skill and reflection-in-action and reflection-on-action (see Ch. 2). Being aware of our own thoughts, feelings and behaviour while we listen, without being distracted by them, can help us to perceive empathetically what clients are trying to convey, even when they do not have the language or capacity to say it explicitly (see Ch. 7). This ability to listen to ourselves and use our inner processes to inform our practice is described by Casement (1985) as the 'internal supervisor'.

Listening

By listening attentively, we shut out extraneous noise and distractions, put aside our own perceptions and thus demonstrate acceptance and respect for those we are with. It is important to choose our words carefully. Using language that is familiar to the patient and avoiding jargon can be very comforting to someone who feels distressed, overwhelmed or confused.

Touch and gestures

Gestures need to be appropriate to the moment but account should always be taken of the person's age, culture, gender and ethnicity. Touching a person's hand when they are looking lost and frightened can be very comforting but in some cultures, men might find it intrusive and inappropriate if a woman does this (see Ch. 1).

In order to be genuine (see Ch. 1), it is important that we do not try to be all things to all people, e.g. by using language or gestures familiar to our clients, but that we would ordinarily find difficult or even offensive. Since we would not usually behave like this, it may seem insincere or incongruent.

Language and paraphrasing

Developing a wide vocabulary is helpful if we are to be able to use the skills addressed below. A rich vocabulary enables us to think of alternative words when a client does not understand. Likewise, if we want to demonstrate we have heard accurately by paraphrasing, knowing a choice of synonyms can help us find the word that exactly describes the person's experience.

That we all bring our personal histories to each encounter influences how we use, as well as perceive, language. Some terms or descriptions that may be commonly used in practice can have very inappropriate connotations for the client and accompanying relatives. An example is instructing a client to position themselves 'on all fours with your bottom in the air', when they need to be in a semi-prone position with their hips higher than their shoulders, usually prior to an examination or treatment. The client is likely to be anxious about the procedure and this undignified position can exacerbate their distress. An alternative instruction could be: 'Please would you kneel, then lean forward and rest on your forearms, so that your hips are higher than your shoulders'. Using terminology that could, at least, be perceived as undignified and, at worst, possibly remind them of very distressing personal experiences such as physical or sexual abuse, can add to their stress and discomfort. Being sensitive to the possible implications of our instructions helps us to offer comfort empathetically, as well as to avoid eliciting distress, however unintentionally.

A warm and gently modulated voice is crucial if we are to demonstrate empathy and to offer comfort. Strident and loud tones are jarring, can be anxiety-provoking and may be perceived as disrespectful.

Body language

Being aware of our body language is essential if we are to demonstrate empathy and offer comfort. People in distress can find that fidgeting or the enthusiastic 'doing' of tasks adds to their discomfort. In order to be there with them, and demonstrate we are listening, we need to be still and quiet. Lack of fidgeting increases the impact of our communication (McFall et al, 1982). It is also necessary to be aware that the position/location of your hands in relation to your body reveals a lot. If, for example, the practitioner or student stands with folded arms while the client is trying to communicate, this might suggest disinterest on the part of the practitioner or student.

Paraphrasing skills

A paraphrase is a shortened statement of what another has said or written. The meaning is not changed but the words are different. Bayne & Tschudin (1998) describe paraphrasing as having two parts: reflection of the spoken words and what is not said but implied.

The value of paraphrasing is that, through the use of this skill, we can demonstrate we are listening attentively and have heard what the other person is telling us. When a practitioner uses this skill, the client can feel supported and understood. Paraphrasing is also a sound way to check and clarify understanding without using questions, which can feel intrusive (see Ch. 5).

Waiting with a patient

You are waiting with a patient in the endoscopy waiting area. She has never been through this procedure before and looks very anxious. She says: 'It's odd, you know. I've had a number of operations and investigations, but they've always been with a general anaesthetic so I've not had to bother about what is going on. This is the first time I've had to be awake while they look inside me. It feels awful – as if I will be right there and involved but not able to do anything to keep control of myself.'

Some issues raised by this scenario:

- This patient has had considerable experience of medical investigations, but never without an anaesthetic. It would be understandable for practitioners to assume that someone with her history would not find yet another investigation any more anxiety-provoking than those she has had before, particularly as this one does not require the intervention and risk of an anaesthetic.

- It is often at the last minute that people disclose their anxiety or distress. Time needs to be taken to listen to them and to respond empathetically. If necessary, procedures need to be delayed to ensure that the patient is fully conversant with what they are about to go through and their consent to the procedure remains valid.

- It is important to explain to the patient that you will share her anxiety with the team so she does not have to worry about repeating it to them. This is important not only for the patient's emotional support but excessive anxiety can lead to physiological changes such as a significantly raised blood pressure. The team needs to be aware of her situation so they are able to decide whether they need to monitor her physiological state in a particular way, or approach the procedure differently, as well as being able to offer her appropriate comfort and support.

Specific principles

- The value of paraphrasing is that it demonstrates to clients that you have understood their story. Clients will tell you how supportive it feels to be heard accurately. Paraphrase demonstrates this and the client thus experiences an empathetic response from you. If, however, what you say is not exactly as the clients meant it, they are able to tell you again of their experience. By offering back what you have now understood by paraphrasing again, you can clarify with them exactly what it is they would like you to appreciate.

- It is important to consider what exactly the patient is telling you. What is she anxious about? It might be lack of control during the procedure and perhaps fear of humiliation, or she might be frightened of pain or of what they might find.

- In this situation the patient should not be rushed into the procedure if there is still any doubt about her awareness of what she is about to face and what the risks might be.

- In order to help the patient to feel heard and supported at the end of the discussion, it is important, whenever possible, to summarize the conversation. This confirms what has been decided or considered and also demonstrates closure of the interaction, which contains the situation and can help the client to feel supported.

Note: A summary is longer than a paraphrase as it covers more content, but like a paraphrase, it addresses the significant issues and keeps the overall meaning of any interaction.

Preparation of self

- Consider what you think the patient might be telling you and what she might be feeling. Try to put these views to one side so they do not influence what you hear.

- Think about what you have noticed about her paralinguistics. Has her voice suddenly become wavering or very soft? This might convey fear or that she is near to tears.

- How will the time, place and manner in which the patient has told her story influence the language you choose and the tone of your voice?

- Think about how you are feeling. You might feel apprehensive that the patient is about to change her mind about having the endoscopy and the fuss this might cause. You might feel under pressure to ensure that she goes ahead with the procedure as she has waited a long time for it; or you might be feeling that you need to get back to the ward and the patient's disclosure will delay this, as it complicates things. Try to put these feelings to one side so they do not influence what you hear.

Environment

- Waiting areas outside theatres can be noisy and busy. It is important therefore to ensure that you notice where you are placed. Ideally you will be positioned away from any thoroughfare in a quiet part of the room.

- Consider where you will position yourself in relation to your patient. You need to be close enough for her to see you and for you to hear each other, but take care not to assume a proximity that might seem discourteous or intrusive.

- If a porter is hovering in preparation to take the patient into the theatre, it might be necessary to ask for some privacy, as you want to talk to the patient. This would also indicate to her that time was being made for her.

Putting the skills into practice

- Position yourself where the patient can see and hear you, but ideally not where you can be overheard. Ensure that you are not standing over her and that you are at eye level with one another. If necessary, find something to sit on.

- Paraphrase what she has said. You might say: *'You're wondering about what it will be like to be awake and involved for the first time during an investigation. The thought of being out of control is a bit frightening.'*

- Allow her to express her anxieties, and explore with her what would help her in this situation.

- Once you have explored together what would be helpful for her in this situation (it might have been that she just needed to express her fears), demonstrate closure of the interaction by summarizing what has been significant to her and how you have agreed to help.

Reflection on practice

Think about a similar situation from your own experience.

- How successful were you in ensuring your patient's privacy?

- How well do you think you did in conveying the essence of what your patient was saying without losing any important points?

- How did the patient respond to you? Sometimes patients express in tears their relief at being heard and understood.

- What did you feel when she disclosed her anxiety to you? How did this influence your choice of words and gestures?

- What, if anything, would you do differently? What are your reasons for this?

- How will you use what you have learned in your future practice?

A distressing interlude

A colleague, Peter, asks if he can talk to you about a situation in practice that he found distressing. You agree and make time to meet him. He says: 'Earlier today I was with a new physiotherapist when she worked with Miss Rushton, who has to learn how to walk again after her hip replacement. The whole process seemed so difficult for her. As she got out of bed I thought she was unnecessarily exposed and I was able to cover her by helping her put on her dressing gown. The physio then started to encourage Miss Rushton to walk. She was very frightened she'd fall again and grabbed on to the table and didn't want to let go. The physio was kind and encouraging, but didn't seem to understand why Miss Rushton was so anxious, although I tried to explain that this was the first time she had tried to walk since her fall. I didn't know how to help and felt very inadequate'.

Some issues raised by this scenario:

- Peter has recognized the need to support and encourage Miss Rushton and how important teamwork is in this situation.
- He seems to have a number of issues that concern him and his practice. He has asked you, as a colleague and a peer, for help to explore them.

Specific principles

- Peter is asking for peer supervision, i.e. the opportunity to explore this situation with someone where the relationship is between equals, as opposed to between individuals with differences in power and authority.
- In this situation, Peter needs time to explore his experience. Agree to meet him when you have adequate time rather than rush the meeting.
- Remember that discussing Peter's practice in this scenario will inevitably mean talking about the patient. Maintaining Miss Rushton's confidentiality is therefore essential. Where you agree to meet must therefore be private so your conversation is not overheard.
- Miss Rushton's physical and emotional wellbeing are paramount. Being unaware of her reasons for being anxious, and therefore unempathetic in response to her fears, might lead to greater resistance to walking and could ultimately hinder her return to independent mobility. For example, she might fear that she will be discharged before she feels ready and able to cope.
- It is important to consider how best to help Miss Rushton to find the courage to try to walk, without being inappropriately controlling or not being encouraging enough out of sympathy for her distress. Peter seems to be aware of this but hasn't said so explicitly.

Empathy and comfort skills

- The skilful use of paraphrase will enable him to feel supported by you. Use questions sparingly as these might sound as if you are interrogating him when he feels sensitive about his practice (see Ch. 5).
- Paraphrasing can help Peter clarify his thoughts and feelings and consider options for future practice.
- It is important to remember how affirmative non-verbal cues such as affirming nods, and sounds such as 'Mmm' can be encouraging to and perceived as supportive of the person telling their experiences.

Preparation of self

- Recognize that Peter is asking for support from you as an equal.
- Consider what Peter's concerns might be, e.g. Miss Rushton's distress, his sense of inadequacy, the physiotherapist's seeming lack of empathy. Try to put these views to one side so they do not influence what you hear and how you respond.

- Think about what you noticed in the way Peter first told you of his experience. Did he seem tense? What was the tone of his voice? Was he relaxed or did he fidget? What did his manner convey to you?

- How did the time, place and manner in which he told you of his concerns influence your decision about how you would explore the issues with him?

- Think about how you are feeling. You might well have been in a similar situation in the past. How might your experience influence how you respond to your colleague's concerns? Because you have been in a similar situation and it raises uncomfortable feelings for you, you might feel the need to soothe Peter's anxieties rather than enable him to explore them with you.

Environment

- Agree when, where and for how long you will meet.

- It is important to find a room that is private and where you are not overheard and are unlikely to be disturbed (see Ch. 6). Ideally, the room is a space that has no particular affiliation for Peter or you, as this can influence subtly how each of you behaves.

- Ensure that you are able to sit comfortably, as this is mutually respectful and encourages a more relaxed interaction.

Putting the skills into practice

- Before you meet, arrange the room so that you can both sit and are able to see and hear each other easily. Ensure, as far as possible, that you won't be disturbed.

- Greet Peter with a smile and position yourself so you are in comfortable proximity to him and can maintain adequate eye contact. Sit quietly and listen attentively.

- Invite Peter to repeat the story by saying something like: *'You had a difficult experience today when you were working with Miss Rushton and the physiotherapist.'*

- When Peter has again described the situation you might paraphrase it as: *'So when you and the physio were helping Miss Rushton to walk, you felt that her anxiety and need for privacy were really not understood by the physio. This meant that you found it hard to know how to intervene effectively.'*

- If Peter replies: 'It wasn't just that I didn't know how to intervene effectively with the physio: it was that I felt so sorry for Miss Rushton because she was so frightened, and the physio just didn't seem to grasp just how frightened she was. Although I was able to encourage Miss Rushton, I felt at a loss as to how to explain this to the physio, especially as I had never worked with her before.'

- You might paraphrase this as: '*Mmm. You wanted to encourage and support Miss Rushton who was frightened, but felt hindered by the fact that you didn't know the physio and didn't want to challenge her, in front of your patient, about her seeming lack of understanding.*'

- Peter might then reply: 'Yes, I really felt uncomfortable because I was torn between not embarrassing the physio and caring for Miss Rushton. It was difficult to know what to say, but talking about it has helped me to see my ethical as well as practical dilemma more clearly.'

- This process of using paraphrase has enabled you *both* to clarify not just how Peter was feeling, but also what his specific difficulties were. In addition, the skill here was to enable Peter to recognize the different dimensions of the situation he was in. By paraphrasing back to him what you heard him tell you, you demonstrate support and empathy.

Reflection on practice

Think of a situation where you have helped someone by demonstrating empathy and understanding.

- How well do you think you did in helping them explore their concerns about their experiences?

- What did their responses tell you of whether they experienced you as empathetic?

- What did you feel when they discussed their experience with you? How did this influence your choice of words and gestures?

- Did they respond as if they felt comforted and supported? Consequently, how did *you* feel?

- What, if anything, would you do differently? What are your reasons for this?

- How will you use what you have learned in your future practice?

APPROPRIATE USE OF TOUCH

'Touch is one of the most universal non-verbal ways of communicating caring' (Sundeen et al 1998: 159). We use it in formal and informal situations to demonstrate human contact such as when we shake hands on first meeting, or when we touch each other in shared amusement. Much of nursing and midwifery practice consists of using touch to carry out technical tasks. How we touch those in our care can convey respect and empathy or, if harshly or inconsiderately done, it can convey lack of care or even disrespect. Using touch skillfully and thoughtfully can convey that you are able to 'be with' your patient (Benner 2001). The scenario below provides an example of the expert interpretation of the need for touch, as is evident in the following account.

The comfort of touch

An acutely distressed woman, who had just learned about the extent of her relative's cancer, was hurrying along a hospital corridor seeking privacy in which to weep. An experienced staff nurse, who did not know her, stopped when she saw her and said: 'You look upset, can I help you? Are you all right?' This compassionate intervention enabled the relative to weep openly and say what had happened. The staff nurse gathered her into her arms, ushered her into an alcove to protect her from prying eyes and allowed her to cry. The woman never forgot how comforting that touch was at a time of acute loneliness.

The rapid assessment of this woman's need, the questions that focused on the immediate situation and the seemingly intuitive use of touch is a sound example of Benner's (2001: 215) description of the expert who is able to engage meaningfully in the situation and rapidly grasp the problem. This intervention was risky, but risk is also in the nature of expertise (Benner 2001).

It is important to note that in a different situation or with different people, such a generous use of touch might well have been inappropriate. If the person does not welcome your use of touch, they are likely to remain stiff and try to back away or extricate themselves. This is the cue to retreat slightly and stay close but not within their personal space.

Meeting a distressed relative

You are going on your break. As you walk through the hospital grounds you see the relative of one of the women on your caseload, sitting on a bench with her head in her hands. As you pass, she takes out a handkerchief and wipes her eyes. She has obviously been crying. You know her partner Tania is at that moment in theatre and that the outcome for their unborn baby is uncertain. Recognizing the relative's distress you approach her and say: 'How are you, Sarah?'

Some issues raised by this scenario:

- Sarah might be apprehensive about how their relationship might be perceived.
- This situation is an example of the importance of unconditional positive regard and empathy, which might be inadvertently overlooked.
- It is also a situation that has the potential for evoking strong emotional responses, both by what this couple is facing, but also from the nature of their relationship. It is therefore one in which emotional intelligence is crucial, so that the practitioner is aware of their feelings about these circumstances, but also very sensitive to Sarah's anxieties and needs.

Specific principles

- As with all communication skills, touch needs to be used with care, i.e. it must always be based on the needs of the distressed person and on the awareness of the practitioner's own motives for intervening. It should *always* be offered respectfully.

- Non-verbal communication is interpreted within the context in which it is offered. How it is offered and interpreted also depends on each individual's personal history and experience (see Ch.1).

- When we use touch, we need to be mindful of culture, age, ethnicity and gender, as these have a significant impact on how our gesture of comfort is received. In some cultures it is unacceptable to be touched at all by people who are not intimates, unless it is in the administration of specific physical care.

- Touching hands is a common form of contact in formal and informal situations. It can be experienced as less intrusive than contact closer to the body.

- In providing midwifery and nursing care, there is often a significant physical component such as when palpating a woman's abdomen or when injections are given.

- How we approach and touch people conveys our sense of their bodily integrity, especially as we frequently need to move into their intimate personal space. This in turn demonstrates our respect and empathy for them.

Preparation of self

- Consider the differences between this scenario and the example given at the introduction of this section. Here you know the person: in the first example, the nurse and the woman were strangers. How do you think this might influence your approach to Sarah and your use of touch?

- As self-awareness is integral to effective communication, consider how your attitudes towards same-sex partnerships might influence the manner in which you intervene. You will want to demonstrate empathy but might be unsure about how best to do this. Be aware of your feelings and how they might influence the way you communicate verbally and non-verbally.

- Consider how to position yourself. If you sit down next to Sarah, you will be more or less level with her, but if the bench is narrow you might find you are too close. You might need to perch on the arm of the bench, or squat discreetly beside it. It is best to avoid remaining standing and leaning over towards Sarah as this can feel intrusive or dominating.

- Will you use touch, and if so, in what way?

- How will your awareness of Sarah's relationship with your patient/client and the place of the interaction, influence the language you choose and the tone of your voice? If Sarah describes herself as 'gay' or lesbian, then it would seem appropriate that you use the same word to describe their relationship.

Environment

- You are in the garden and so in an exposed place. It is important to try and make the space around you personal and private, e.g. by positioning yourself in a way that excludes onlookers or other people who might want to sit on the same bench. One way of doing this is by facing Sarah and having your back to the surrounding grounds.
- Bearing in mind that your break time is limited, you will need to decide how you will manage the time available to be with Sarah.

Putting the skills into practice

- Approach Sarah and greet her by name. If necessary, remind her of your name. Position yourself so you can shut out any interested onlookers.
- You might say: *'I can see you're upset. Is there anything I can do to help?'*
- Wait for her reply. Unless she communicates clearly that she doesn't want to talk to you, you might ask if you can sit down.
- Sit facing her but in a position that doesn't crowd her and is not too direct: sideways on to someone often feels like a less direct or dominant position.
- Say something that acknowledges her difficult position and how distressing it is. You might like to say how difficult it is to wait while her partner (use her name, Tania) is in theatre. This is offering Sarah the opportunity to talk.
- When she starts to unburden herself, think of her need for physical comfort and the use of touch.
- Be guided by your own inner feelings about what seems an appropriate non-verbal response to Sarah's distress, as well as by her posture and behaviour. For example, she might lean closer to you, indicating the need for an arm around her shoulders. On the other hand she might lean forward and talk to you with her face in her hands to hide her tears but not necessarily to shut you out. A brief touch on her shoulder as opposed to an arm around them, might seem more appropriate than no touch at all. As touching hands is a common form of contact, and can be experienced as less intrusive than contact closer to the body, you might feel easier reaching out and touching her hand, if she isn't covering her face.
- After she has unburdened herself you might need to address the time, as you might be due on the ward soon. You might say: *'I need to go back to the ward now. Is there anything I can do to help when I get back?'* If there is, undertake to do it if at all possible. Ask her how she is feeling now. Offer to help again if she and her partner need it or refer her to expert help if appropriate.

Reflection on practice

Think of a situation where you have tried to comfort someone in distress.

- What prompted you to intervene? Were you tempted to pass by?
- Think about your thoughts and feelings as you approached the person. How did your emotional intelligence prompt your self-awareness and the

awareness of the circumstances in which you found yourself? What thoughts did you have as you approached the distressed person?

- How did this awareness influence your responses? How did it influence your use, or not, of touch? Consider if you would have responded differently if the person were in a similar position to Sarah in the scenario. How might this influence your responses?

- Consider what you did to ensure the person's privacy. How successful were you in enabling them to explore their worries?

- How did you perceive the person's response to your care? How did you end the encounter?

- What, if anything, would you do differently? What are your reasons for this?

- How will you use what you have learned in your future practice?

AWARENESS OF CULTURAL DIFFERENCES IN THE EXPRESSION OF DISTRESS

Culture and communication are addressed in Chapter 1. This section will focus on cultural differences in the expression of distress.

In order to provide comfort we need to be aware that we all respond differently to distressing experiences. As culture has a significant impact on our verbal and non-verbal cues (Sundeen et al 1998) it can be difficult to attribute meaning to the non-verbal cues people give (Grasha 1995). In some cultures it is not acceptable to express uncomfortable emotions, so distress might be managed through stoical silence, whereas in others, people might need to verbalize their suffering loudly.

Reactions to distress

Ms Leinster, a 40-year-old single woman whose father is a British army officer, is on your ward. She has just been told she has cancer. She sits quietly, looks very subdued and says little. At handover you are told that she is 'coping very well with the news'. From the end of the ward you notice that she is very still and has refused the offer of afternoon tea. The patient in the next bed has her family with her and they are all crying noisily. You go up to Ms Leinster and ask how she is.

Some issues raised by this scenario:

- The patient might have been brought up in a culture where it is important not to display overt emotions. Just because she is quiet and not weeping openly does not mean she is not distressed.

- The handover report demonstrates a cultural interpretation of the patient's response.

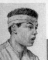

Specific principles

- It is important to be aware of your own assumptions about the 'acceptable' way to express distress. This will help you avoid making inaccurate assessments of how troubled a person might be.

- Although people express distress differently, it is important to offer comfort even though they might choose to refuse it.

- The use of ritual during a major life event such as after the death of a loved one, can provide people with a source of protection and support in their community (Hoff et al 2009). As practitioners we need to accept people's different rituals and manifestations of distress in order to support them.

- Whatever the religious or cultural background of the client, it is always crucial to treat their expressions of distress with respect (Neuberger 1994).

- It is important always to see those in our care as individuals. When we demonstrate willingness to learn about others' cultures and religious customs we demonstrate acceptance and respect. This willingness to accept people as they are is very comforting to the distressed person and their loved ones (Neuberger 1994).

Preparation of self

- Drawing on what you know from experience and the literature about people's responses to distressing news, consider how your patient might be feeling. Recognizing the processes of coming to terms with distressing news can help you to empathize and can inform how you respond.

- Think about what you noticed about your patient's demeanour. Did she seem on the verge of tears or was she withdrawn but polite? What did her manner convey to you?

- Be aware of how you are feeling. You might feel very distressed that someone in your care is having to face such a frightening diagnosis. How might your feelings influence how you open the conversation with your patient? How might they be manifest in your non-verbal cues?

Environment

- In a ward it is often difficult to ensure patients have privacy. In this case, the patient is quiet and subdued. If she wants to, it is important to offer to go elsewhere if she seems reluctant to talk in an open place. Drawing the screens can help.

- Ensure that you make time to be with the patient. Rushing an interview with someone in distress can limit the comfort they might draw from your care. Explain to your colleagues so that they do not interrupt.

Putting the skills into practice

- Approach your patient's bed quietly. Position yourself where you can see each other but do not crowd her by coming too close.

- Greet her by name and ask how she is. You might like to say how sorry you were to hear about her diagnosis. Ask her if she would like to talk about it at all.

- Offer to go somewhere more private. If she chooses this option, ensure that the room is private, you are both seated comfortably and there are tissues if needed.

- It is likely that, as she is reticent, she might not say very much at first, if at all. Just because she doesn't say anything does not mean your concern and presence aren't wanted or comforting.

- Sitting still and quietly with the patient, even if she says little, can be comforting to her. This form of 'being there' (Benner 2001: 30) has been experienced by some people as graciousness in times of deep distress. It is the privilege of nursing and midwifery.

- If your patient does want to talk to you, be guided by her. Here the use of paraphrase can help her to feel supported and heard. It also allows her to lead the conversation. Listen quietly and attentively and be aware of your body language.

- When the patient appears comforted and it is appropriate to close the conversation, ask if there is anything she might like you to do before you leave and offer an example such as, asking if there is anyone you could contact for her?

- Clarify with the patient what you will record in her nursing notes. Any information that needs to be shared with the team should be entered.

Reflection on practice

Think about a similar situation from your practice where your client's display of distress was different from what you would have expected.

- How did your feelings before you approached your client influence what you said and your non-verbal cues?

- How did the different manner of expressing distress influence your responses during and after the interview? You might have felt sad but honoured that the client confided in you; or at the end you might have left feeling hopeless and despondent.

- How successful were you in ensuring your client's privacy?

- How effective were you in allowing your client to lead the conversation and so express her feelings in her own way and time?

- How empathetic and comforting do you think you appeared? What in your client's behaviour leads you to think this?

- What, if anything, would you do differently? What are your reasons for this?

- What have you learned about culture and people's assumptions about the expression of distress? How will this influence your practice in future?
- How has your understanding of the significance of emotional intelligence informed your reflection? How do you think this understanding will enable you to develop your practice?

ENSURING PRIVACY AND DIGNITY

Chaperoning a patient

An 80-year-old woman with abdominal pain is being seen for the first time in Outpatients by a male physician. She has never been to the hospital before and appears very nervous. You are asked to chaperone her while the physician examines her. As part of this process he does a rectal examination.

Some issues raised by this scenario:
- The patient has to face strangers in an unknown environment. She has an undiagnosed problem and is likely to be nervous about the outcome of her investigations.
- Not only is the environment strange and the situation potentially frightening, but she does not know the doctor or you.
- Part of the examination includes a rectal examination, which can feel intrusive and embarrassing.
- The patient is an older woman and the doctor is younger than she is. She might have different views from you about proper conduct between an older woman and a younger man in these circumstances (Le May 1998). It is important to ensure that your presence is supportive and promotes the dignity of the older person (Nursing and Midwifery Council 2009, Royal College of Nursing 2008).

Specific principles

- In this scenario the patient has never met any of the people involved in her care. She is also in an unfamiliar environment. It is important to help her feel at ease by introducing yourself and introducing her to the doctor.
- People of different ages have different roles in life. This often means they have different values and 'prefer interacting with those whom they perceive in some way as equals' (Le May 1998: 94) in shared life experiences rather than try and overcome cross-generational differences in experience. It is important to take this into account when building a relationship with this patient. It might be helpful to explain that you are working 'with' her and engage her in the partnership by explaining how important it is for you that she lets you know how best to assist her during this consultation. The gender

difference as well as the age difference between the patient and the doctor might add to her embarrassment.

Preparation of self

- How do you think the patient might be feeling during the process of visiting Outpatients and having a medical consultation? How will your thoughts inform your practice?

- How will you introduce yourself? How will you introduce her to the doctor? What touch do you think is appropriate during these introductions?

- How will you engage her as an equal partner in her care? Consider the age differences between you.

- Is gender an issue here? If it is an issue in the development of this professional relationship, how do you think it might influence the maintenance of her privacy and dignity in this situation? If a female nurse is available, it is important to ask your patient if she would prefer to be chaperoned by a woman. If however the doctor is female, and you are male, explain this to the patient and check whether she is happy for you to be with her.

- Consider what you will say to the patient during the procedure and after it is over. So as not to interrupt inappropriately or confuse the patient, be sure to ask the doctor to explain everything as he/she goes along.

- How will you ensure she is comfortable during and after the examination? Consider how you will use touch. Holding her hand during the procedure is more formal and remaining near her head rather than observing the procedure is important.

Environment

- Ensure your patient has sufficient time to undress. Rushing to take clothes off can feel undignified and, as an older adult, she might take a little longer.

- Ensure that the curtains to the examination room are closed and that the door is shut.

- Check that a modesty sheet is available for the patient so she is not unnecessarily exposed.

- Ensure that all the equipment needed for the examination is readily to hand so the patient does not experience preventable delays while she is waiting or already in the process of being examined. This can add to her anxiety.

- Ensure that she has somewhere to hang her clothes and a discreet place to put her underwear.

Putting the skills into practice

- Clarify with the doctor how he likes to conduct the examination and what he explains to patients during investigations.

- Greet your patient by name and introduce yourself. Offer your hand to shake if this seems appropriate. It is a formal way of touching someone and can convey warmth and respect.

- Explain your role and how you would like to work with her, i.e. try and engage her in a partnership with you by showing that you are equals in this endeavour. You both want to ensure that her visit runs as smoothly as possible.

- Ask her to let you know how you might assist her during the consultation. Demonstrate empathy by recognizing that this is an unfamiliar situation and she might find that stressful.

- The physical component to this examination is likely to feel intrusive and embarrassing. How we help to maintain this patient's dignity and privacy is a crucial part of demonstrating empathy and offering comfort, particularly as this examination will move into her intimate personal space. A supportive touch on her hand or arm might help her to feel at ease.

- You might say: 'Coming to see a new doctor is often difficult, especially when we have never had an examination like this before. (Name) so that you feel as supported as possible, it is important to me that you let me know how I can help you while you are here. I will be staying with you throughout, so please let me know if there is anything worrying you.'

- Introduce the doctor by name to the patient using his full name. Then introduce the patient to the doctor using her full name and title. This too demonstrates respect for her dignity.

   Note: The order of this process may be culturally determined.

- Check whether she would like you to remain during the initial discussion with the doctor. If she does, position yourself where she can see you and where you can respond to her needs should she ask for your assistance.

- Before the examination, ask her if she needs any help to undress, explaining what clothing she needs to remove. Show her where she can put her clothes.

- If she needs help to get on to the couch, assist her with this. She might just need a hand to support her as she uses the steps to get up on to the couch. A firm hand grip is supportive and can be reassuring.

- When the doctor begins the examination, stand at the top of the couch where she can see you and ensure she is not unnecessarily exposed. During the rectal examination, offer to hold her hand. Encourage her to express any feelings or discomfort. You might say, 'Please do let us know if you feel discomfort or pain, because Dr (Name) would like to cause as little discomfort to you as possible.'

- At the end of the examination, when the doctor has left the room, offer her a tissue to wipe away any lubricant and show her where to wash her hands.

- Ask her if she needs help, and if necessary, assist her to dress. Allow her sufficient time for this, *as well as to compose herself,* so that she doesn't feel rushed and undignified.

- After the doctor has finished the consultation, ensure that she has made arrangements to get home and can find her way out of the department. Offer a positive statement about having been with her – you might say, *'I am pleased to have met you, (Name)'* when you say goodbye.

Reflection on practice

Reflect on a similar situation where you have chaperoned a patient of a similar age, whom you had not met before.

- As you are younger than your patient, consider your thoughts and feelings when you introduced yourself. How did these influence what you said and your non-verbal cues?

- How effective were you in engaging your patient as a partner in care? What indicators have you for your conclusions?

- How successful were you in working in partnership with both the doctor and the patient while ensuring you maintained your role as patient/client advocate? What observations of the processes of working together have informed your conclusions?

- How successful were you in ensuring your patient's/client's dignity and privacy?

- What, if anything, would you do differently? What are your reasons for this? How will this influence your practice in future?

PROVIDING EMOTIONAL SUPPORT FOR PEOPLE EXPERIENCING INTENSE FEELINGS

Dealing with an angry outburst

You are working on the postnatal ward. Mrs Ailsa Griffiths, has been waiting all morning for the neonatologist to examine the baby prior to their discharge home. Her husband Selwyn has come to collect them. He had been assured by the staff, that his wife and baby would be ready for discharge on his arrival to the ward. This was of particular importance to him because he had already had several penalty charges for exceeding parking time in the hospital car park. He is very angry and shouts so loudly in the ward that everyone present can hear. He then storms away to his wife's bed area and slams various items on the bedside locker. You realize he has been very stressed because his wife had been admitted antenatally and had had to stay in hospital until she had their baby. You seek him out to offer support.

Some issues raised by this scenario:

- Selwyn is obviously distressed. Could his outburst have been foreseen?

- The outburst in such a public arena is significant. It is important to consider what the reasons for this might have been. What messages might this convey?

- What effect might his outburst have had on any onlookers such as other women in the ward, and staff? How could these be addressed?

Specific principles

- Find out the reason for the situation, i.e. why his wife and their baby have not yet been seen by the neonatologist. There might have been unavoidable reasons for this unfortunate situation, but it is also important not to offer to promise to solve the difficulty if your commitment cannot be fulfilled.

- It is important to be aware of your own assumptions about the 'acceptable' way to express and manage intense emotions. All individuals do this in their own way. For example, sometimes people find it easier, and perhaps safer, to do so publicly as a means of managing their feelings.

- When people express intense emotions, it can spark intense feelings in us, perhaps of anxiety, fear or indeed feelings similar to theirs. When we recognize how we feel in these situations, we can manage our feelings and put them aside, in order to help the person in our care.

- Be aware that after a person has had an emotional outburst, they might feel they have lost their dignity. It is important that as practitioners we do all we can to offer care that supports a person's dignity (Royal College of Nursing 2008). In situations where the person's outburst might elicit in them a sense of having lost their dignity, we need to be respectful so as not to exacerbate their uncomfortable feelings or distress.

- Because of the intensity of the situation, you might feel you want to remove yourself or respond defensively, rather than go to Selwyn. Being aware of this possibility and, if you personally are not in any imminent physical danger, it is appropriate to go to and stay quietly with the person. Consider getting someone more experienced to deal with this situation. (For details on violence in healthcare, see Hoff et al 2009 and Wykes 1994).

- Position yourself where Selwyn can see you and, if necessary, where you can touch him. Avoid fidgeting and position yourself where you can maintain eye contact. Standing while he is sitting down might be perceived as threatening. Be aware that intruding on his personal space can be perceived as threatening and/or challenging.

- If possible, suggest that he sits down with you, as this can help reduce the physical manifestations of any further intense outbursts because when we sit we are more limited in our movements as well as more inclined to relax.

- Offer him the opportunity to tell you about his feelings. This can help alleviate the intensity of his emotions, and be cathartic. By being empathetic and not avoiding his distress, you offer the opportunity for acceptance, as well as the containment of what can feel like overwhelming and unmanageable feelings.

- It is also important to remember the containing nature of time limits. Once Selwyn is calmer, let him know that you will soon have to close the conversation. Give him some warning of how much longer you can stay and listen before you actually take your leave. Try as far as possible to keep to your commitment. Setting time limits is usually experienced as containing, especially as you haven't succumbed under the weight of his emotion. Offering to talk to him again after the consultant has seen their baby demonstrates that you are still willing to be there for him and accept him, despite his outburst.

- If any other women or visitors comment on what has happened, you might say, 'The situation is all right now.' Be absolutely sure that Mr and Mrs Griffiths' privacy and confidentiality is maintained by not discussing any of the details of the situation.

Note: It is also important to recognize the limits to your role in the containment of intense feelings and, if necessary, refer people on to more specialist services such as counselling or psychiatric services.

Preparation of self

- What did you feel when you witnessed Selwyn's outburst? You might have felt frightened by the intensity of his feelings, sorry that he was so stressed and perhaps angry with him for disrupting the quiet of the ward. How might your feelings influence how you approach Selwyn? How might they be manifest in your non-verbal cues?

- Think about whether it might help you to talk to a colleague for a few minutes before you go and talk to Selwyn. This can help you clarify your thoughts, feelings and strategies for helping him and his wife.

- Ailsa is likely also to be disappointed and let down by the neonatologist and the ward team. She has been in hospital longer than she expected and is looking forward to going home with her baby to her husband. How will you include her in the conversation? What might you say to ensure that you recognize that, as a couple and as new parents, they might share similar feelings about this prolonged wait to go home?

- Consider how he might be feeling underneath the anger. He might feel let down by the neonatologist and feel that the doctor and the ward team have failed him and his family. He might also be feeling powerless to do much to change the situation.

- Think about what you noticed about his non-verbal cues. Was he making violent gestures? Perhaps he seemed let down, but also frustrated. What did his overall demeanour convey to you?

- Think about how much time you have available to help Selwyn. Keep this in mind so that his feelings don't seem to take over the rest of your work. How will you open the conversation with him?

- When you approach him, what will you say? How will you position yourself?

- Consider what options you have for following up the cause of his anger. When and how will you offer them to him and his wife?

- Consider how and when you will end the conversation.

Environment

- Selwyn has sought space to express his intense feelings by going to his wife's bedside area and slamming things about on the locker. Consider how you might approach him there to speak to him while recognizing his need for dignity and privacy.

- Consider if it is appropriate to stay there or move somewhere else like the office. However, as a number of people have overheard this outburst, going somewhere else might feel very exposing to him, particularly if he begins to feel embarrassed by his behaviour.

Putting the skills into practice

- Consider how you are feeling. Acknowledge your feelings and put them to one side. If you are apprehensive about how you will cope, it can help to discuss this with a colleague for the few minutes before you go and talk to Selwyn.

- Wait a few moments to allow Selwyn to gather himself. This is also an opportunity for you to compose yourself if you felt discomfited by his outburst.

- Ensure that you make time to be with him so you can show empathy with him about this situation. Rushing the interview might contribute to his feeling of not being heard or valued and powerless in the face of the staff and the institution.

- Go to Ailsa's bed area and ask him by name if you might talk together about the situation. Wait for his response. He might take a little while to acknowledge your approach. Try and initiate collaboration. When you are with Selwyn and Ailsa ask if they would like you to close the curtains or talk in a private room such as the office, to ensure their privacy.

- You might say: '*I recognize there are issues concerning the delays you have been experiencing that we need to talk about.*'

- Depending on his response, you might like to say how sorry you are about what has happened.

- Try to arrange chairs beside the bed so that you can all sit in comfortable proximity with level eye contact. If you go to an office, arrange the chairs in a similar way. Avoid sitting behind the desk as this can be construed as setting up a barrier between them and you.

- Ask Selwyn to tell you about his anger. If it seems appropriate and Ailsa has come to the office with you, invite her to say how she feels about the situation. Sit quietly with them without fidgeting or demonstrating any anxiety you might feel.

- Listen quietly and attentively to the emotions expressed, the language they use and also to what they *do not* say (see Jacobs 2004). Be aware too of your body language. 'Being with' (Benner 2001: 50) can be comforting, even if Selwyn says a lot and seems not to want to listen to you, because you have not run away from his intense feelings.

- Be guided by him in how to encourage him to talk. The use of paraphrase can help him feel he is being listened to and supported (see above). Questions can feel controlling if not sensitively used (see Ch. 5). Bear in mind that underneath his anger there might be a range of conflicting and difficult feelings about his wife's early admission and the subsequent delays in seeing the doctors, culminating in this instance, which are hard to identify and express.

- When he appears calmer, encourage a partnership between him and his wife and yourself, by exploring with him options for resolving the situation now.

- Before ending the encounter, ask Selwyn how he is now, say how pleased you are that he has talked to you and clarify what you have agreed can be done to deal with the situation.

- Before closing the conversation, ask him and his wife if they would like to return to the ward or wait in the relative privacy of the day room. This can support Selwyn, allow for quiet conversation between the couple as well as help to address any curiosity among other people on the ward and staff. Ask him too if he would like you to be with him while he speaks to the neonatologist.

- Before leaving Selwyn, say you will let him know how things are progressing, then close the conversation.

- Record in Ailsa's notes exactly what happened, what you agreed to do to resolve the situation and by when. Share your decisions with the midwifery team.

Reflection on practice

Think about a situation in your nursing or midwifery experience when you have had to deal with an angry outburst.

- What did you feel at the time? You might have felt frightened by the intensity of the feelings and angry about the disruption it caused. How did this influence what you said to the person and your non-verbal cues?

- How did you feel during and after the interaction with the angry person? You might have felt embarrassed about the cause of the outburst, but relieved that you were able to demonstrate empathy in such a difficult situation. How did your feelings influence your practice?

- How successful were you in ensuring privacy and dignity for all involved, while at the same time allowing the angry person to express their feelings in their own way and time?

- How empathetic and comforting do you think you were? What leads you to think this?

- What, if anything, would you do differently? What are your reasons for this?

- What have you learned about helping people to express and manage their intense emotions? How will this influence your practice in future?

References

Bayne, R., Tschudin, V., 1998. Listening: some basic qualities and skills. In: Bayne, R., Nicolson, P., Norton, I. (Eds.), Counselling and Communication Skills for Medical and Health Practitioners. BPS Books, Leicester, pp. 41–50.

Benner, P., 2001. From Novice to Expert. Excellence and Power in Clinical Nursing Practice. Prentice Hall, New Jersey.

Casement, P., 1985. On Learning from the Patient. Routledge, London.

Christensen, J., 1993. Nursing Partnership: A Model for Nursing Practice. Churchill Livingstone, Edinburgh, pp. 115–142.

Golman, D., 1998. Working with Emotional Intelligence. Bloomsbury, London.

Grasha, A.F., 1995. Practical Applications of Psychology, 4th edn. HarperCollins, New York.

Hoff, L.A., Hallisey, B.J., Hoff, M., 2009. People in Crisis: Clinical and Diversity Perspectives, 6th edn. Routledge, New York.

Jacobs, M., 2004. Psychodynamic Counselling in Action, 3rd edn. Sage, London.

Kadner, K., 1994. Therapeutic intimacy in nursing. J. Adv. Nurs. 19, 215–218.

Le May, A., 1998. Empowering older people through communication. In: Kendall, S. (Ed.), Health and Empowerment Research and Practice. Arnold, London, pp. 91–111.

McFall, M., Winnett, R., Bordewick, M., 1982. Non-verbal components in the communication of assertiveness. Behav. Modif. 6, 121–140.

Neuberger, J., 1994. Caring for Dying People of Different Faiths, 2nd edn. Mosby, London.

Nursing and Midwifery Council, 2009. Guidance for the Care of Older People. Nursing and Midwifery Council, London.

OUP, 1989. Oxford English Dictionary, Oxford University Press, Oxford. Online (accessed 28 March 2009).

Rogers, C., 1957. The necessary and sufficient conditions of therapeutic personality change. J. Consult. Psychol. 21, 95–103.

Royal College of Nursing, 2008. Campaign on Dignity (continuing). Online. Available at: www.rcn.org.uk/__data/assets/pdf_file/0003/191730/003298.pdf (accessed 22 April 2009).

Sundeen, S.J., Stuart, G.W., Rankin, E.A.D., Cohen, S.A., 1998. Nurse–Client Interaction: Implementing the Nursing Process, 7th edn. Mosby, St Louis.

Wykes, T. (Ed.), 1994. Violence and Health Care Professionals. Chapman & Hall, London.

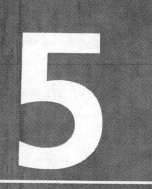

5

Interview and assessment skills

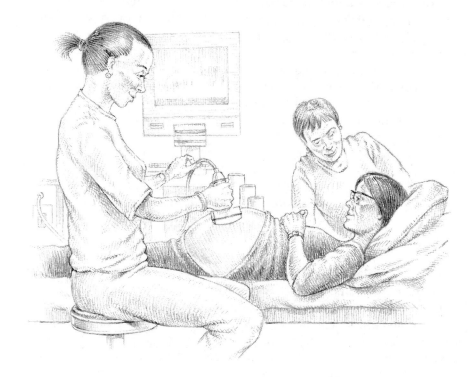

INTRODUCTION

Interviewing and assessment form the foundations of all our conscious and unconscious interactions with others, whether they are formal, such as in an interview for a job, or informal, such as when we meet a newcomer to a tutorial group. We make conscious decisions on the information we glean from effective interviewing, e.g. determining the needs of the patient or client. These decisions are based on our knowledge and experience, but they are also based on unconscious experiences, that will influence our perceptions of the situation.

Physical messages that we observe such as the woman's or patient's physical condition or our colleagues' non-verbal cues, influence how we respond in those particular circumstances. Paralinguistics, language choice and voice modulation are clues to how the other person might be feeling. We need, therefore, to be aware of what we have observed and how we choose to respond when we are interviewing and making an assessment. The purpose and focus of the interview and assessment are more readily evident in formal situations, but might be less clear when, e.g. we are reviewing a patient's care plan or a woman's birth plan.

Assessment is the first stage of the nursing and midwifery processes. It forms the foundation of all the care to follow. As the nursing and midwifery processes are dynamic, care is adjusted according to the changing needs of those in our care. In order to do this successfully, we need to assess patients' and women's needs continually.

This chapter explores the skills we use when we interview others. It addresses how we make effective assessments and the skills we use to develop further our professional relationships and deliver care. The skills which will be considered are: questioning skills, explanation skills and giving information to relatives.

PRINCIPLES

In order to interview and assess effectively, there are a number of principles we need to apply. The purpose of each interview and the focus of each assessment need to be clear, both to you as the practitioner, and to those who are involved in the situation with you. In order to develop a partnership with the others in the interview, it is important that you engage them in the process and encourage their co-operation. The feelings of all involved influence the interview and assessment processes. It is key, therefore, to a successful interview, that you are aware of how you are feeling and of your body language. It is equally important to observe the non-verbal cues of those you are interviewing. These can give you clues to how they might be feeling.

Where you have a number of women or patients to care for during a shift, you need to decide whose needs take priority, thus who you will interview and assess first. When and where you hold the interview may influence its process. It is important, therefore, to make the environment as friendly and private as possible.

If time is limited, as in an emergency, the attention of the others involved needs to be drawn to this. By doing so, you can help them to understand the reasons for quick interactions, such as asking a number of closed questions when assessing a newly admitted woman in labour.

You need always to be sensitive to the diversity of those in your care. All of us come to interviews with our own understanding of appropriate behaviour in the circumstances. Our cultural, social, personal and professional heritages will influence how we perceive others as well as how we behave in relation to them and in that situation. These factors will also influence the interactions of our colleagues and clients, as well as those occurring in informal interactions (see Ch. 1). Cultural difference is evident in subtle ways as well as in the more obvious such as race, language and religion. Think too about issues such as age, gender, occupation and which part of the country a person comes from. English dialect can be confusing even to those whose mother tongue it is. 'Tea' to one person might mean the early evening meal, but to someone else it might mean a cup of tea. You can demonstrate sensitivity by observing the language others use and choosing words that are as unambiguous as possible. Take care when you use metaphors and idioms, as these are usually culturally specific. An example is the term 'to spend a penny' which means 'to pass urine'. This term is commonly used in certain groups, but it might not make sense to people who do not remember when it cost 1 penny to use the public toilets!

Avoid questions beginning with 'Why?' These are apt to sound accusatory or critical. 'Why did you tell the doctor you were worried about Mr Patel?' can sound as if you think your colleague has done something wrong in discussing concerns about the patient with the doctor. It would be preferable to say: 'What were your reasons for telling the doctor you were worried about Mr Patel?' This question will elicit information about Mr Patel's condition as well as the rationale for talking to the doctor caring for him.

QUESTIONING SKILLS

We use questions for a variety of reasons, such as to show we are listening, to encourage others to disclose information or to join in the conversation as a group discussion, and to explore and clarify situations. The skilful use of questions is integral to effective interviewing and assessment.

Closed questions

These are questions to which there is only one answer, such as 'Yes' or 'No'. They can be used when you want specific information. They limit explanation and can help ensure that interviews keep to the point. They are therefore also useful on occasions when a short answer is appropriate such as when you are in a hurry, or when the person you are addressing is breathless or acutely distressed. Examples are: 'Are you alright?', 'Are you still in pain?'

Open questions

Open questions differ from closed questions as they allow for a wide range of answers. You will find them useful for exploring issues and seeking wider perspectives. When we ask open questions we allow the other person to describe their experiences, feelings or understanding. Examples are: 'How are you feeling?', 'What happened?'

Open focused questions

These are questions that are open, but focus on specific areas. They are useful if you wish to address particular issues or experiences. Examples are: 'What was your reason for choosing the birthing pool for your labour and delivery?' 'What was your experience of being with the occupational therapist in the community?'

Assessing a distressed pregnant woman

Mrs Angela McBride is a 30-year-old Irish woman who was admitted to your ward last night. She seems to be miscarrying her first and much longed-for baby and is due to have an ultrasound scan to assess the state of her pregnancy. She is quiet but obviously very distressed. You are asked by the Midwife in Charge of the antenatal ward to find out how Mrs McBride is feeling before she goes for an ultrasound scan.

Some issues raised by this scenario:
- Mrs McBride is facing a deeply distressing life event – the possibility of losing her baby. You know she is distressed and will need sensitive care. It would be helpful for you to know more specifically how she feels so you can be perceptive in meeting her needs for support.
- Mrs McBride's knowledge of her situation needs to be assessed.
- Finding out how she feels about having a scan and what its results might be will enable you to offer her appropriate reassurance and information.
- The value of a scan and how it is actually carried out needs explaining.
- When people are very distressed, they often need to be given the same information on a number of occasions.

Specific principles

- When interviewing and assessing someone's needs it is always important to state your reason for requiring the information.
- Open questions give a wide range of possible answers; closed questions can identify exact information.
- Closed questions are especially important in situations where complicated or long answers would be too demanding for patients and women in

your care, such as when they are in a lot of distress through pain or breathlessness.

- As only limited answers are required, closed questions can be experienced by the person being interviewed as controlling because they cannot expand on their experiences, e.g. when you are taking a nursing history.
- If you use a mixture of open, closed and open focused questions skilfully, you will be effective in interviewing and assessing the needs of others and the situations in which you are practising.

Preparation of self

- Think about how you feel about Mrs McBride's situation. Have there been other occasions where patients or friends have lost pregnancies and you have cared for them?
- It is understandable that you too might feel distressed about Mrs McBride's situation. How do you think you can use the awareness of your feelings to help her?
- Think about how you are feeling about asking Mrs McBride about her feelings. You might feel apprehensive about intruding or concerned that you might say the wrong thing.
- Consider what sort of information you need from Mrs McBride in order to offer her appropriate support.
- What is the best way for you to gain this information? What skills will you use? If you intend to use questions, what will they be – open, closed or open focused?
- How will you open the interview?
- What do you hope Mrs McBride will gain from the assessment of her needs?
- Think about what you have noticed about Mrs McBride's demeanour. Is she withdrawn, tearful or putting a brave face on things?

Environment

- Ideally this should be private and out of others' hearing. However, this can be difficult to attain on an open ward but closing the curtains partially or completely provides some privacy.
- If you are talking to a patient or client and assessing their needs in a public place, e.g. the street after an accident, try to make space around the person, which effectively 'shuts out' any onlookers. One way to do this is to turn your back on onlookers and keep the person shielded as far as possible by your presence. This can be done by the way you position yourself and any equipment you might have with you.
- If you want to sit on a patient's or client's bed, it is important to ask permission. Unless they have a private room, the bed is usually the only exclusively personal space that patients or women on the maternity unit have when they are in hospital.

Putting the skills into practice

- What you observe about Mrs McBride will guide you as to how to open the interview so you can assess her needs for support and information, as well as for physical care.

- It is helpful to approach her bed quietly as she seems distressed. Consider whether it will be sensitive to sit on her bed or pull up a chair.

- Greet Mrs McBride and introduce yourself if this is the first time you have met her. A beaming smile does not seem appropriate, although a warm facial expression will show her you are interested in meeting her and caring for her.

- If this is the first time you have met, it might help the interview to be relaxed if you engage her with a short social interaction like commenting on her bedside plants or get-well cards.

- You might use an open question like: 'How are you, Mrs McBride?' Depending on her answer and her emotional response, you can decide where to sit.

- She might well respond tearfully or in a similarly distressed manner. It is very important to sit quietly and 'be with' the patient (Benner 2001: 50).

- If she is weeping, avoid platitudes like: 'It's going to be all right', as clearly you cannot know that. A sensitive comment acknowledging her distress like, *'I am so sorry you are having such a difficult time'* demonstrates empathy (see Ch. 4).

- It is advisable to wait quietly until Mrs McBride has gathered herself and seems able to talk to you.

- If she is very distressed you might pass her a tissue and/or ask her if she would prefer you to come back in a few minutes. Be sure to make eye contact with her, even if only fleetingly, to show you are not evading her distress. However, making eye contact is culturally very specific, so it is important to be aware of different cultural norms. Watch for signs that eye contact is too intimate (i.e. if the patient looks uncomfortable) and gauge when to look away (see Ch. 1).

- Be aware of how you are feeling as 'strong feelings are contagious' (Platt & Gordon 2004: 57). This self-awareness can help you to avoid being caught up in your own emotions that the situation has aroused in you: it will also enable you to listen empathetically.

- When she is ready, you can then assess her knowledge about the need for having a scan, by asking in a gently modulated voice an open focused question such as, *'What do you understand about why the doctors have arranged for you to have a scan?'*

- Address any questions she might have and clarify anything she does not understand or has not been advised about. Explain the process to her, outlining the procedure: when, where and how it will happen, who is likely to do the scan and whether she will be chaperoned. Ask her if she would like anyone to be with her (e.g. husband, partner, relative or friend).

- Ensure that you follow local procedures and if necessary inform the relevant department that someone will be accompanying Mrs McBride.

Reflection on practice

Think of a situation from your experience where you have assessed a distressed patient or client.

- What were your feelings during the assessment of the person in your care's needs? How do you think they influenced the way you responded?

- How did the person respond when you went to assess their needs?

- If you were able to sit quietly with them, what was their response? What interventions seemed to help the most?

- If relatives or friends were present, how did you support them? If you included the person's partner in the assessment, how did you do this?

- How did other staff members help you with this assessment? What feedback do you think the nursing team needed in order to give the patient sensitive and appropriate care? How, when and where did you give it? What did you document in the care plan?

- What would you like to have done differently? What observations of yourself and the responses of those in your care prompted you to consider these changes? How will you use this learning in future practice?

EXPLANATION SKILLS

Explanation enables us to clarify our thinking, helps others to understand the reasons for our decisions and is essential in the teaching of others. Patients and clients might need information about a variety of issues: a first time mother will probably need to know how they will be cared for during labour; an ill person might need help to understand the nature of their illness; students and colleagues might need help to understand a new technique or policy. Effective use of questions enables you to assess how much the person knows and understands. Set aside enough time and start by clarifying the person's understanding of the topic. Assess the person's physical and emotional state as these influence how much they can absorb and for how long. Use an interpreter if necessary (see Ch. 7).

Give a brief overview of the topic, starting with what the patient or client already understands, and avoid using jargon and giving them too much information at once. Talk logically through the topic, linking important issues coherently. Allow time for them to consider what you have said and to ask questions. Check understanding of the key points regularly by asking the person to tell you what they have understood. Open focused questions are useful here.

Finish with a clear summary and follow-up with written details and contact numbers as appropriate. If the explanation is required because the person's condition has worsened, it is important to be honest and not give false hope. Your tone of voice, choice of words and manner all need to be empathetic.

In the following scenario, the woman needs information about the significance of being sent to a specialist unit, what this entails and when she is likely to know about the wellbeing of her baby.

Explanation skills

Mrs McBride is aware of the need for a scan but does not understand why she has to go to a specialist department – the Early Pregnancy Assessment Unit – as up until now, she has had scans in the main X-ray department.

Some issues raised by this scenario:

- Mrs McBride's fears about the implications of going to a specialist unit
- Whether or not she will be able to be accompanied by you and/or her husband
- When she is likely to be told about the outcome of her scan and by whom.

Preparation of self

- Identify equipment/aids that might be needed. In this instance, a leaflet on the Early Pregnancy Assessment Unit and the value of ultrasonic scans in pregnancy would be appropriate.
- Ensure you are thoroughly versed in what it is you intend to explain. What procedures are followed when a woman seems to be miscarrying in early pregnancy and needs a scan? Identify the limits to your knowledge and authority to pass on information.
- Choose a private area where you will not be overheard if at all possible.
- Reflect on the type of relationship you have with the person to whom you are giving the explanation.
- Decide on the essential pieces of information and how they are interrelated.

Environment

- Wherever possible, this should be private and out of earshot. In an open ward, pull the curtains partially or completely around the bed for privacy, if this suits the patient. If Mrs McBride is in a side room, close the door with her consent.
- If you feel it is appropriate to sit on Mrs McBride's bed, it is important to ask her permission.

Putting the skills into practice

- Take into account Mrs McBride's emotional state. When people are distressed and anxious, it is difficult for them to take in information and so it might need to be repeated.
- Clarify a starting point by finding out what the patient already knows. You might ask, 'What do you know about having a scan?' This is particularly

important when the person is distressed as it helps them to focus on the relevance of the information to their situation.

- Provide a context for the explanation that the other person understands. This helps to reassure them that the issue is relevant to them personally.
- Talk logically through the information, from the agreed starting point to the end, linking the information so that it makes a coherent whole.
- Check understanding regularly by asking the other person to paraphrase what they understand and by using open focused questions.
- If the person does not understand, re-frame the information using age-, culture-and situation-appropriate metaphors. Use adjectives and descriptions to which the other person can relate. This is where cultural awareness in the use of metaphors is important (see Ch. 1).
- When you have finished your explanation, ask the other person to repeat what they have understood.
- Ask the other person what questions they might have. Avoid asking the closed question, 'Have you any questions?' It is better to ask something like, *'Is there anything else that you would like me to clarify?'*
- Where possible, provide written information to support your explanation, e.g. a leaflet on ultrasound scans.

Reflection on practice

Consider a situation from your practice when you gave an explanation about treatment to someone in your care.

- What aspects of your explanation went well? What are your reasons for thinking this?
- How coherent was your explanation of the need for the treatment and what it entailed? What would you like to have done differently?
- If you had to clarify aspects more than once, what were the reasons for this? Perhaps you might have worded your questions differently or used shorter sentences. In situations where patients are anxious or distressed, as with Mrs McBride, they might have found it hard to take in everything you were saying.
- How did the patient seem at the end of the explanation? What are your reasons for thinking this?
- How will what you have learnt from this reflection influence the way in which you give explanations in future?

GIVING INFORMATION TO RELATIVES

Giving information to relatives about the wellbeing of those in our care is an everyday and essential part of effective communication in nursing practice. The Nursing and Midwifery Council is clear that we need to be able to do this without breaching patient confidentiality (Nursing and Midwifery Council 2008) but we also need to avoid seeming 'cagey' or withholding, thereby offending people who have genuine concerns about their loved ones. Relatives are also among the people to whom we offer care. This is most obvious when the news about their loved one is worrying or likely to cause distress. Always ensure that what you tell relatives is accurate and appropriate and that you have the knowledge and authority to do so.

Checking the identity of enquirers

A student nurse is working in a rehabilitation centre for patients who have suffered some form of brain injury. The student knows most of the patients well as he has cared for many of them over the preceding weeks. A young woman, whom the student had not previously met, introduces herself as Marcia Goldsmith and asks: 'Nurse, please would you tell me how my father, Mr Pringle, is getting on?'

Some issues raised by this scenario:

- The identity of the woman and her relationship to Mr Pringle, who she says is her father
- Whether or not Ms Goldsmith is known to the other centre staff, either as a documented next-of-kin in the patient's records or as someone they have met and talked to in the past
- Whether or not Mr Pringle has identified her as his daughter and what he would like her to know about his situation and progress
- How the student is going to clarify these issues before sharing information with Ms Goldsmith.

Specific principles

- As professional practitioners we have a responsibility to keep confidential all the information we have about clients and patients. Sharing information about those in our care must be guided by professional ethics and the Code of Professional Conduct (Nursing and Midwifery Council 2008).
- Patients and clients have a right to privacy (Human Rights Act 1998). The ethics and protocols of giving information about people in our care to relatives differ from those governing information-sharing with colleagues. There are specific protocols (e.g. Chief Medical Officer of England 1997) for information-sharing across professional disciplines.
- Sharing information needs to be justified, appropriate and proportionate to the situation, auditable and necessary (Human Rights Act 1998).
- The support patients and clients receive from their relatives varies from person to person, their particular family relationships and culture. The information we share about them must always reflect the requests of those in our care, not the wishes of their family and/or friends.

- A holistic approach to care for patients and clients does however mean that we need to offer support and understanding to their relatives and friends.

- It is essential always to be very clear that patients or clients consent to your sharing information, exactly what information you might share and with whom.

- Take care not to make assumptions about who those patients or clients regard as their relatives. Same-sex couples might name their partner as their next-of-kin and not want their blood relatives to know anything about their condition. It is important to be aware that this might upset other relatives but the person's wishes must be respected.

- If people request information about a patient or a pregnant woman in your care, it is important to be sure of the identity of the person enquiring and whether or not the patient or client wants them to be kept informed (see Ch. 7).

- In situations where there is a risk of violence to the patient or client, e.g. when a woman has been admitted with injuries as a result of domestic violence, it is **crucial** that you do not expose the patient to further risk by disclosing information such as their whereabouts. Always check in these situations whether or not the patient consents to your disclosing this information and to whom. Significant skill is required here to avoid giving information in such a way as to show that the victim is in your care. For example, refusing to give information about a person in your care on the grounds of confidentiality is an admission that the person is in your care.

- Whenever possible, share information in a private place, out of earshot of others. Avoid corridor conversations.

Preparation of self

- Be absolutely certain that you know what the patient or client consents to your disclosing and to whom.

- Be sure you know the identity of the people asking for information before you disclose anything about the person in your care. In this situation, you need to consider how you intend to ensure that Ms Goldsmith is who she says she is.

- It is important that any information you disclose is accurate and appropriate.

- Decide what you are going to say and what words you will use. Avoid using abbreviations like 'obs' for observations.

- Ensure that you use easily understandable words rather than technical terms, as these can confuse and worry relatives, especially if they are anxious or unfamiliar with medical and nursing and midwifery terminology.

- How are you feeling about talking to Ms Goldsmith? Do you have the necessary knowledge and experience? Would you prefer a qualified staff member to speak to her instead, or to be with you while you do so?

Environment

- The environment in the centre should be one where people in your care and relatives feel safe, psychologically and physically.
- If Ms Goldsmith has not been there before she might feel intimidated or anxious in a strange place, especially if there is a lot of activity or rehabilitation equipment in the environment where you meet.
- Your manner of greeting will be important to help Ms Goldsmith to feel valued and her father well-cared-for.

Putting the skills into practice

- To ensure you know that Ms Goldsmith is Mr Pringle's daughter, you might need to ask another member of staff to confirm her identity, or you might need to ask Mr Pringle if he would like to see her and confirm her identity for you.
- This can be done in a friendly and assertive manner by saying something like, *'It is nice to meet you, Ms Goldsmith. I'm sure you understand that as we've never met before, it's important that your father or another nurse who knows you introduces me to you before we discuss his progress.'*
- Clarify what she wants to know and clarify exactly what Mr Pringle is happy for her to know. This you can do by asking him and/or looking at his records.
- If Mr Pringle does not want her to know anything other than that he is 'alright', you need to be sure you can say this without seeming to be withholding, especially if Ms Goldsmith has a lot of questions.
- Decide exactly what you are going to say, where and how.
- If it is appropriate, share the information with Mr Pringle present, so he can explain his situation and progress to his daughter himself.
- Take care to share information in a private place. Shut the door. If this is not possible, draw curtains or move away from people who might be able to overhear your conversation. If possible, offer Ms Goldsmith a chair to sit down, and sit down too.
- If the news might cause distress, it is **crucial** that it is shared in private and Ms Goldsmith has enough time and space to take in the information, ask questions and express her feelings. **Never** disclose disappointing or bad news in a public arena.
- Arrange the space so that if people look in, her facial expressions and non-verbal cues are not easily viewed from the outside, e.g. position her chair facing away from the window.
- Always make time to share information. This might mean asking Ms Goldsmith to wait while you finish what you are doing before you go and speak to her. When the news is distressing, making enough time is crucially important.
- If you cannot find a private space to talk to her, place yourself between her and any onlookers so that you make a secluded space that discourages others

from interrupting you. One way of doing this would be to find a corner and stand with your back to the room with Ms Goldsmith facing you. **Note:** It is never acceptable to give anything other than positive information in a public place.

- Allow time for Ms Goldsmith to ask any questions she might have and, before ending the interview, check that she is satisfied and has nothing else to clarify.
- Be sure to show that the interview is over by taking your leave cordially. You might stand up and offer to shake her hand.
- If the news has been bad, it is caring and very important to ensure that she has some sort of support getting home and/or when she gets home, if this is at all possible. If necessary, check whether it is possible to arrange for someone to collect her.

Reflection on practice

Think of a situation when you have had to check the identity of someone who was enquiring about a patient/client on your ward.

- How did you feel about checking the identity of the person before you gave any information about their relative/friend?
- What aspects of your information-sharing went well? What are your reasons for thinking this?
- How effective was your explanation of the need to check the person's identity? What would you have preferred to have done differently?
- If you had to explain the situation and the patient's or client's progress more than once, what were the reasons for this? Perhaps you might have worded your information differently or used shorter sentences. Perhaps the relative was more anxious than you realized and might have found it hard to take in everything you were saying.
- How did the relative seem at the end of the interview? What are your reasons for thinking this?
- What did you find most challenging in that situation? How will you use what you have learned from this reflection in your future practice?

GIVING INFORMATION OVER THE TELEPHONE

Dealing with an aggressive caller

A man telephones the ward where you are a student nurse. He asks loudly if his wife Mrs James is there and how she is. He does not give you his name and when you ask for it, he becomes abusive and says: 'Don't be ridiculous! I've told you I am Mrs James's husband and I have a right to know how she is!' You are aware that Mrs James has described her marital status as 'separated'.

Some issues raised by this scenario:

- Mrs James has said she is separated and therefore you **must not** assume to disclose any information about her to her estranged husband, unless she advises you otherwise.
- As with all other enquirers, he needs to be treated with respect but Mrs James needs to have the final say as to who is informed about her progress.
- He is aggressive. This can be a sign of acute distress caused by fear for a loved one but it could also be due to concern that he might not be able to find out about her because of her choices to exclude him for reasons of her own.
- If Mrs James is happy for information to be disclosed to him you need to verify his identity (see below).

Specific principles

- The principles of confidentiality as stated in the Nursing and Midwifery Code of Conduct (Nursing and Midwifery Council 2008) and patient or client choice apply to the disclosure of information concerning them to relatives enquiring about their progress.
- If anyone requests information about someone in your care, it is important to be sure of the identity of the person enquiring and whether or not the patient or client wants them to be kept informed (see Ch. 7).
- As before, always ensure that what you tell relatives and enquirers is accurate, appropriate and that you have the authority to disclose the information.
- The information we share on the telephone must always reflect the wishes of those in our care, not those of their family and/or friends.
- It is essential always to be clear that the patient or client consents to your sharing information, exactly what information you may share and with whom, whether on the telephone or in person.
- On the telephone it is easier to miss situations where there is a risk of violence to the person in your care. These are as **crucial** as they are in face-to-face enquiries. You **must** ensure that you do not expose the patient to risk by inadvertently disclosing information such as their whereabouts. Note that this takes forethought and skill.
- **Always verify** the identity of the enquirer as far as possible. If necessary, ask for a telephone number which you can check against next-of-kin details and/ or which you can use to telephone the enquirer back.
- If you are unsure as to the identity of the enquirer refrain from disclosing **anything** about the patient, including that they are in your unit or on the ward. It is important to take care not to do this inadvertently by saying something that infers their condition or implies that they are on your unit.
- Whenever possible, share information in a private place, out of earshot of others. If this is not possible when using the telephone, keep your voice low so others are less likely to overhear your conversation.

Preparation of self

- Take time to notice how you are feeling in response to the caller's attitude. You might be taken aback by his vociferousness or indeed frightened by his behaviour.

- When we feel strong emotional responses, especially when we find ourselves in unexpectedly intense situations, we can respond immediately 'from the heart' without thinking. Here the old maxim 'count to 10' can help us draw breath before saying anything.

- Consider how the caller might be feeling. This can help you choose words which demonstrate empathy by acknowledging his anger (Lindenfield 1992), rather than those which might alienate the caller.

- Speak calmly without raising your voice and in measured tones. Avoid raising your voice in response.

- Say something like: *'I understand that my not discussing anything concerning our patients with you, can be very frustrating and therefore you sound angry.'* Avoid platitudes like: 'I hear you sound angry,' or 'I know how you feel.' None of us can 'know' exactly how someone else feels, as we are all unique and respond to situations in our own way. Likewise, it is not possible to 'make' someone feel the way they do, although it is possible to understand how they **might** be feeling in a given situation.

- Reflecting back (Clark 2003) to the caller what they are saying, can help them to feel you empathize with their situation, and thus they may calm down. Be wary of using the 'fogging strategy' (Clark 2003) as that can fuel the person's anger and frustration, particularly if it sounds as if they are being fobbed off or condescended to, however inadvertently.

- Keep in mind what you know about the behaviour of abusive intimate partners and relatives. If this is the case, be **very careful** not to disclose that Mrs James is on the ward.

Environment

- Think about the environment you are in. Is the telephone in the middle of the ward, or are you answering it in the office?

- If you are in a public area, who is likely to overhear you? Would it be better to take the call in the ward office?

Putting the skills into practice

- Keep your voice calm and well-modulated.
- Ask for the caller's name and address him by it.
- Offer empathy and encourage cooperation by saying something like, *'I can appreciate you are concerned, Mr X, but I am sure you will understand that for reasons of patient confidentiality, I cannot let you know who is on the ward.'*

Note: Do not ask the caller to hold the line while you enquire, because this action will disclose to him that she is on the ward.

- Avoid being drawn into a battle of wills, by repeating your statement courteously and firmly, but recognizing all along that he is obviously concerned.
- **Do not** ask for contact details by which you can ensure he is contactable by his estranged wife, as this will disclose her whereabouts.
- End the conversation by thanking him for calling and for his understanding and say goodbye.
- After you have ended the call, go and talk to Mrs James and let her know Mr X had called asking after her. Explain that as you were aware she was separated from her husband and you did not know whether or not she wanted him informed about her whereabouts and condition, you did not let him know she was on the ward.
- Clarify with Mrs James who she would like informed about her presence on the ward and offer to help her telephone Mr X if that is what she would like to do.
- Ensure that you record Mrs James's wishes and this incident in the nursing records and that you notify your colleagues at handover.

Reflection on practice

Think about a situation from practice when you have had to deal with an aggressive caller on the telephone.

- Consider how you felt when the caller became aggressive and impatient with you. What were your gut reactions? These are 'as valuable as theory' (Ash 1995: 26). How did these feelings affect your thinking?
- When you recall what you actually said, were there any particular points in the interactions that resulted in the caller being mollified?
- What aspects of the conversation did you deal with well? What aspects of this conversation could you have dealt with better? What are your reasons for thinking this?
- How do you feel you dealt with the caller's distress?
- How do you think what you have learnt from this situation will influence your practice in future?

Informing relatives of an emergency admission

A patient is admitted to your ward following a fall in which he fractured his ankle and he now needs surgery. You need to ring his wife and inform her of his admission.

Some issues raised by this scenario:

- Consider whether you have the skills to carry out this task or need supervision from someone else. If you do need to ask someone more experienced, try to listen to what is said so that you can gain experience.

- Your patient is likely to be anxious about not having contacted his wife as his admission was an emergency. He is also likely to be very concerned about how his wife might respond to the news.

- Anxiety can make it difficult for patients to think clearly. Your patient might therefore have difficulty remembering where his wife is and how to contact her.

- The patient's wife might well be quite shocked by your telephone call and the news you are giving her.

Specific principles

- The principles of confidentiality and patient choice addressed above apply to the disclosure of information concerning them to their relatives, even when they have asked you to contact their next-of-kin.

- It is important to check with the patient exactly the name and contact details of his wife and what he is happy for her to know about his circumstances and condition. If necessary, write down exactly what he would like her to be told.

- Make the call as soon as possible after the patient has been admitted.

- Take into account the effect your call and the news is likely to have on the recipient. This patient's wife is likely to be shocked and need reassurance.

- As it is most unlikely that your patient will have any toiletries and pyjamas, ask him what he would like his wife to bring in. Make a list of what he needs. Remember to suggest things like reading matter that might make the time pass more quickly.

- If the patient's wife asks you about his progress be sure to use language that is reassuring but honest. Do not disclose anything more than the patient has agreed for you to say.

Preparation of self

- Consider how you feel about contacting a stranger to advise her of her husband's accident. How do you think your feelings might interfere with how you will break the news that he is in hospital?

- Choose beforehand the words you will use to describe your patient's circumstances and condition to her. If necessary, write out your opening sentences or list a few phrases to help you through the conversation.

- Be prepared for a relative who might be anxious, unco-operative or unwilling to help.

- Think about what you might say in these circumstances.

Environment

- As always, it is important to think about the environment you are in. Ensure as far as possible you are out of earshot of people other than the healthcare team. If you can, use the office telephone.

- Try to ensure that you are unlikely to be interrupted when you are making the call; finish immediate tasks and close the office door when you make the call.

Putting the skills into practice

- Before you pick up the telephone, check that you are sure of the wife's name and title. Check also that you have the correct number and the list of your patient's requirements.

- When the telephone is answered, introduce yourself with your title and place of work and ask to speak to the woman concerned by her full name, i.e. title, first name and surname.

- Be sure to reassure the person receiving your call that there is no cause for her to be unduly worried.

- Ask her name before you disclose anything.

- Explain clearly the circumstances of your call. You might say something like, *'There is nothing to worry about unduly, but unfortunately your husband (name) has been admitted to our ward (name) at (name of hospital). He has asked me to let you know he fell and broke his ankle today and will need an operation later, but that he is alright and you're not to worry.'*

- Answer all the wife's questions as honestly as you can in a well-modulated tone and with empathy. Acknowledge that this is probably a shock for her. Reassure her as to your patient's progress and condition.

- Listen carefully for any feelings she might be expressing in her comments and questions. Demonstrate empathy by paraphrasing briefly what his wife is saying and by not answering too quickly. Pausing like this also gives you time to think about how you might respond sensitively as well as demonstrates that you are listening (Nelson-Jones 2006).

- His wife is likely to want to visit and bring him his pyjamas and toiletries. When it seems appropriate, tell her he has said what he would like her to bring. List clearly all the things your patient has asked for. Ask his wife to clarify what she has understood.

- Ask her if she has any messages for her husband or questions for you.

- Before ending the conversation, ensure she knows the ward details, its whereabouts, how to reach the hospital and how to contact you. Advise her of how to get there and repeat your name and the ward telephone number.

Reflection on practice

Think of a situation when you have had to telephone an unsuspecting relative to give news about a patient.

- What did you think and feel before you made the telephone call? Well-prepared, rushed, ill at ease? How did you deal with your feelings?

- How well did you establish a professional relationship with the relative? Review what you actually said. Were there any particular points in the interactions that helped you to build a rapport with them?

- What aspects of the telephone call did you deal with well? What are your reasons for thinking this?

- Were there any aspects of this conversation that you could have dealt with better? What are your reasons for thinking this? Your feelings about the call might help you reflect on this aspect of your practice.

- How do you think what you have learnt from this reflection will influence your future practice?

References

Ash, E., 1995. Supervision – taking account of feelings. In: Pritchard, J. (Ed.), Good Practice in Supervision. Jessica Kingsley, London, pp. 20–30.

Benner, P., 2001. From Novice to Expert: Excellence and Power in Clinical Nursing Practice. Prentice Hall, New Jersey.

Chief Medical Officer of England, 1997. The Caldicot Committee: Report on the Review of Patient-identifiable information. CMO, London.

Clark, C.C., 2003. Holistic Assertiveness Skills for Nurses. Springer, New York.

Human Rights Act, 1998. Home Office, London.

Lindenfield, G., 1992. Super Confidence. Thorsons, London.

Nelson-Jones, R., 2006. Human Relationship Skills, 4th edn. Routledge, London.

Nursing and Midwifery Council, 2008. Code of Professional Conduct. Nursing and Midwifery Council, London. Online. Available at: www.nmc-uk.org/aArticle.aspx?ArticleID=3056 (accessed 13 March 2009).

Platt, F.W., Gordon, H.G., 2004. Field Guide to the Difficult Patient Interview, 2nd edn. Lippincott Williams and Wilkins, Philadelphia.

Further reading

Stevenson, C., Grieves, M., Stein-Parbury, J., 2004. Patient and Person: Empowering Interpersonal Relationships in Nursing. Elsevier Churchill Livingstone, Edinburgh.

6

Assertiveness, advocacy and negotiation skills

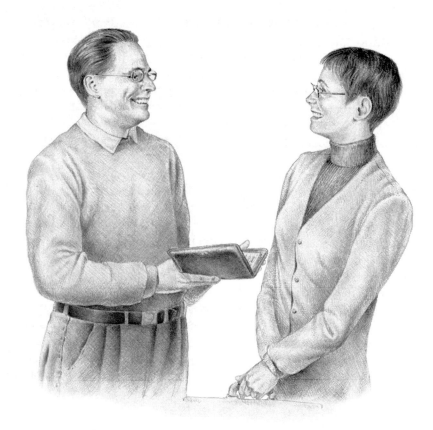

INTRODUCTION

Nursing and midwifery take place within organizations and require effective communication with everyone involved, in order to ensure competent and safe practice. This chapter addresses some of the important skills that practitioners need to develop so that a good standard of care can be provided. These skills include: using assertive communication; acting on behalf of another if appropriate; and negotiating activities. While assertive communication facilitates compromise and negotiation, there are occasions when this is not the best option and examples of alternative strategies are also explored. Assertiveness also involves being clear about professional boundaries and the chapter concludes with a discussion about boundary-making skills.

ASSERTIVENESS

Assertive communication is the key to communicating important messages to others (Fig. 6.1). It also helps individuals to stand up for their rights and, when appropriate, the rights of others (e.g. advocacy). As a practitioner within a professional team, using assertiveness skills is an essential component of working in a proficient manner. There are a number of key principles that describe the concept of assertiveness. Essentially, these principles identify types of behaviour, attitudes and feelings that influence how we interact with others. Rakos (1991) provides a thorough discussion of the various theoretical perspectives that underpin assertiveness.

Assertive messages are clear, succinct and respect the self-esteem of the person being addressed, as well as that of the speaker. Such messages may be used to articulate an opinion that is different from that of the majority, reveal a lack of knowledge or skill, or express a concern. There is a risk to the individual's self-esteem, however, that the other person(s) might not respect this information and that the response might be aggressive or dismissive. The underlying philosophical belief regarding assertive behaviour is that of 'I'm OK – you're OK' (Harris 2004, Berne 1975).

Using assertive behaviour in the form of clear and focused communication can enhance the quality of our personal and professional relationships. Assertive behaviour might not always be the most appropriate response; e.g. where there might be a high risk of personal injury, a passive or manipulative approach might be best. Assertive behaviour might be difficult for an individual for a number of reasons, including cultural norms, lack of information, lack of awareness, lack of support or lack of appropriate skills.

The preferred style for handling conflict and decision-making varies across cultures. Those from individualist cultures (see Ch. 1) were found to use strategies that maximized their own interests at the expense of others, while those from collectivist cultures used a negotiating style that took the interests of others into account (Oetzel 1995, Witte & Morrison 1995). In collectivist cultures harmonious

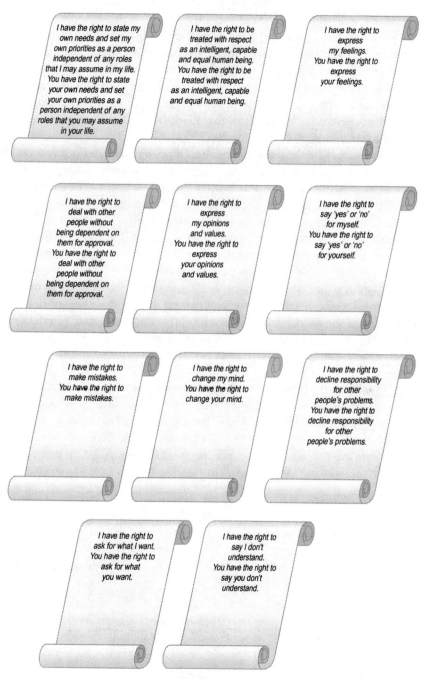

I have the right to state my own needs and set my own priorities as a person independent of any roles that I may assume in my life. You have the right to state your own needs and set your own priorities as a person independent of any roles that you may assume in your life.

I have the right to be treated with respect as an intelligent, capable and equal human being. You have the right to be treated with respect as an intelligent, capable and equal human being.

I have the right to express my feelings. You have the right to express your feelings.

I have the right to deal with other people without being dependent on them for approval. You have the right to deal with other people without being dependent on them for approval.

I have the right to express my opinions and values. You have the right to express your opinions and values.

I have the right to say 'yes' or 'no' for myself. You have the right to say 'yes' or 'no' for yourself.

I have the right to make mistakes. You have the right to make mistakes.

I have the right to change my mind. You have the right to change your mind.

I have the right to decline responsibility for other people's problems. You have the right to decline responsibility for other people's problems.

I have the right to ask for what I want. You have the right to ask for what you want.

I have the right to say I don't understand. You have the right to say you don't understand.

Figure 6.1 Bill of assertive rights (adapted from Dickson 1982 and Bond 1986).

relationships are considered essential and it might be felt to be inappropriate to place great emphasis on assertive behaviour, which by definition focuses on the individual. In addition, people from Asian cultures are identified as tending to prefer not to use the word 'no', therefore 'yes' might mean 'no' or 'perhaps'. It is therefore essential to seek clarity when in conversation, in order to ensure that information, instructions and implications have been understood. For an informed discussion on cultural factors that might affect the western principle of assertiveness, see Kim (1995) and Singelis (1994).

Paying attention, listening and minimizing fidgeting increase the impact of the communication (McFall et al 1982). An upright position with good eye contact is desirable; this means adopting intermittent and comfortable eye contact, which is neither a glare nor gives the appearance of staring. Body movements should be steady and smooth and an audible, clear and appropriately modulated tone of voice used. Fluency while speaking is a feature of effective assertive communication. Rakos (1991) found that the use of inflection, e.g. changing tone or placing emphasis on an important part of a statement, was also very effective. If you are highlighting a discrepancy or challenging an opinion, it might be useful to consider whether you are the best person to have this conversation and whether you and the other person are in a receptive frame of mind, physically and psychologically. For example if either of you have just finished a long shift, tiredness or fatigue might adversely affect perception, cognitive ability and/or reasoning.

In any given situation there are choices as to how one can respond. The style of responding can be passive, manipulative, assertive or aggressive. A brief explanation of these behaviours follows. (For a more detailed discussion, see Seaward 2009, Bond 1986, Paul 1985 and Dickson 1982). Examples of verbal responses from the different perspectives are provided in Box 6.1. In addition, analysis of transactions is facilitated by considering Berne's (1975) ego state

Box 6.1   Examples of verbal responses

In the following responses, the same example has been used to illustrate the differences in verbal presentation. As well as the verbal statements that represent the various responses, you need to consider the body language, tone of voice and emphasis that may be used.

The nurse has just completed a ward round with a doctor. The doctor is about to leave the ward and has forgotten to request investigations for one of the patients that has been seen. The nurse wishes to draw this omission to the doctor's attention.

Passive behaviour (I'm not OK – you're OK)

The nurse's speech is high-pitched or quiet, there is minimal eye contact and the sentence lacks fluency and consistency. There is also some hesitancy.

Continued

Box 6.1 | **Examples of verbal responses—Cont'd**

Nurse: Doesn't say anything to the doctor, but complains to other colleagues about the doctor's inefficiency once the doctor has left the ward

or

Nurse to doctor: *'I'm really sorry to bother you, I could be wrong, but did you want Mrs Jones to have an ECG. I wonder if you could possibly, er ... complete the request form?'*

Manipulative behaviour (I'm OK – you're not OK, but I'll let you think you are)

The nurse speaks softly, possibly seductively or louder than the circumstance warrants. There is likely to be intermittent or continued eye contact and possibly reduced personal space. Once the task has been completed this personal space is likely to be increased.

Nurse to doctor: *'You're usually so good about these things, would you like me to get the request form for Mrs Jones ready for you to sign?'*

Aggressive behaviour (I'm OK – you're not OK)

The nurse's body language might be very rigid or overactive, with the tone and speech short and abrupt, the statement perhaps being totally unexpected by the doctor. There might also be a hint of sarcasm and impatience. Eye contact might vary from a firm glare to none at all, signalling a disregard for the other person. The statement is more of a demand than a request.

Nurse: *'You've forgotten to complete the form for Mrs Jones. You doctors are always forgetting to do these things and we have to keep phoning you to come to the ward. Can you do it now please, and then we can send it off.'*

Assertive behaviour (I'm OK – you're OK)

The nurse gains the doctor's attention and establishes eye contact. Speech is clear, fluent and non-accusatory, and the tone of voice is moderate.

Nurse: *'I think you've forgotten to write a form for Mrs Jones. Would you like to do it now or will you be coming back to the ward later to do it?'*

---

model (parent, adult and child), a description of which appears in the glossary (Appendix 1). The different styles of responding available to us have both verbal and non-verbal characteristics, e.g. body language and tone of voice.

Passive behaviour

This behaviour is based on a belief, that in a given situation we consider ourselves to be less worthy when compared with others. This might be because we do not feel as capable as the other person generally or in a given situation. In certain circumstances this might be the safest option; however if this is the general pattern of behaviour, it is likely that self-esteem is compromised and the individual is not living to their full potential. When this position is used, verbal presentation tends to include the use of long sentences that lack focus and contain statements that discount the value of the individual's opinion. There are also frequent apologies.

A major disadvantage of always communicating in this pattern is that others might interpret passive behaviour as a lack of interest or knowledge. This might lead to people becoming frustrated in trying to involve someone who does not appear to be interested or able to participate. Equally, people might believe that the person is incapable and therefore they might not be included in decision-making. Either way, passive individuals are left feeling less worthy than their colleagues, and fear, anger and/or sadness are common feelings and can lead to a self-fulfilling prophecy (see Appendix 1).

Manipulative behaviour

As children, we have all learnt different ways to get what we want. As adults, this might have developed to include encouraging others with the use of flattery or flirtation (which is not genuine) towards an action that meets our desired outcome. This activity is sometimes referred to as 'stroking someone's ego'. In a group, for example, this might result in an individual thinking that they have made a decision when what has actually happened was that they were coerced (unconsciously) into making the decision. This strategy will only work however if the other person is open or receptive to the 'hook' that has been dangled. In transactional analysis (e.g. Stewart 2007, Berne 1975), this could be referred to as an ulterior transaction.

A manipulative strategy may sometimes be used in order to 'save the face' of another person, who might otherwise feel embarrassed if their lack of knowledge or skill were exposed. One of the disadvantages of taking the responsibility for 'saving the face' of someone else might be that one's own knowledge and skills go unnoticed and resentment might build up. It also means that the person being manipulated does not get an opportunity to develop their knowledge and skills, if they are always being rescued. Feelings such as anger, guilt and embarrassment need to be taken into consideration before deciding whether or not to use this style of communicating in a given situation.

Manipulation can be considered a negative pattern of behaviour if the feelings and needs of the other person are disregarded, or if others are treated as objects to fulfil the needs of the manipulator. However, the use of a manipulative style of communication is the preferred way of interacting in some cultures. This is not seen as a means of deceiving another person, rather a manner of approach that is less direct than in western cultures.

One way of assessing the style of communication is to consider whether or not the thoughts and feelings of the other person have been taken into account. It may be appropriate to provide feedback to the sender of a message about the impact of their style of communication in order to make them aware of its effect on you.

Aggressive behaviour

When we interact from this position, we have assumed that our rights are the only ones that matter; we will also find it difficult to acknowledge any mistakes that we have made, since this is a position of superiority in comparison with others. Fear, anger and anxiety might be the underlying feelings that result in verbally attacking others, using sarcasm, employing threatening tones and blaming. While responding in this way might be a one-off, repeated experiences and observations by patients and other members of the team might result in a tense working environment and strained communications.

Assertive behaviour

This perspective acknowledges the rights and responsibilities of oneself and others, as well as the strengths and weaknesses that are a part of being human. Communication is open, honest and personalized; and compromise and negotiation are key features of the interactions. The main advantages of communicating in this style are that individuals experience the satisfaction of expressing themselves as well as listening to the needs of others. However, individuals who have a preference for communicating in any of the above ways might find it frustrating (the manipulator), frightening (the passive person) and irritating (the aggressor) when in communication with an assertive person. This is because they are likely to be offered the opportunity to discuss and negotiate their concerns in an understanding manner. For example, imagine trying to maintain an argument with someone who is demonstrating an understanding of your concern and offering to help solve the problem.

Assertive communication skills are used to express one's thoughts, feelings, needs, wants, beliefs and opinions and, while focused on oneself, an integral part of assertiveness is the recognition that others also have the right to do the same. Negotiation and compromise are therefore key features of being assertive. Box 6.1 gives examples of different verbal responses.

Being assertive to ensure patient safety

There is a patient in the recovery area who has had an invasive procedure. You have agreed to collect them. Having received a handover from the nurse or midwife, you are unhappy to take the patient back to the ward.

Some issues raised by this scenario:

- As a registered nurse or midwife you will be expected to collect patients or women following procedures that require sedation, general or local anaesthetic.
- There might be occasions when you do not feel competent to undertake this activity. Patient and client safety might be compromised if you

accept a task for which you are not adequately prepared. It is therefore essential that you inform the appropriate person if this is the case. The Nursing and Midwifery Council (2008a) in the UK outlines practitioners' responsibilities to those in their care by stating that they must be competent to practice and have been educated and trained for the purpose of their professions.

Specific principles

Strategies to consider in such situations include: how to say 'no'; how to negotiate an alternative; how to use effective self-disclosure; and the importance of using all senses to gather information.

Prior to collecting a patient following a procedure, ensure that you are familiar with the condition the patient is likely to be in, on return to the ward. Ensure that the bed area the patient will return to is prepared and any equipment that is needed is available, assembled and in working order. You might need to take equipment with you to ensure the person's comfort and safety during the journey back to the ward. For example, a receiver, airway and swabs or tissues might be useful if the person in your care is feeling nauseous or if they wish to expectorate. Specific equipment such as an abduction wedge pillow (following total hip replacement) or clip removers might also be required. Check the local policy.

Gather appropriate information from the staff member who has asked you to collect the patient (e.g. patient details, the procedure performed), particularly if you are not familiar with the person and the procedure.

Preparation of self

- What is the basis of your concern? Do you have factual information (e.g. vital signs, visual observations, etc.) or is this an intuitive feeling? (Atkinson & Claxton 2000)
- How are you going to get the information necessary to allay or confirm your concern? For example, what are the person's vital signs? What information do your visual and aural observations give you about the amount of drainage, colour of the patient, breathing pattern and respiratory sounds? (Reed 2003)
- Do you have sufficient information to ensure clarity of the statement you intend to make? If not, consider using open, closed and open focused questions to get the information that you need.
- It might also be appropriate to ask yourself what the implications might be if you decide not to be assertive in this situation.

Environment

- It is important to take time to consider the appropriateness of the environment in relation to the conversation that you intend to have. While the person's eyes may not be open, the sense of hearing is the first to return following an anaesthetic and they may become anxious if they overhear your concerns.

- How close are the other patients in the recovery area? How are you going to maintain confidentiality during this conversation?

Putting it into practice

- If you consider that some of the information you have received is inconsistent, or you cannot make the necessary links between what you are being told and what you observe the person's condition to be, seek clarification in a non-accusatory way. For example:
  - **Recovery Practitioner**: *'The wound was oozing quite a bit but I have changed the dressing and the patient is fine now.'*
  - **Registered Nurse/Midwife**: *'Yes, the wound does appear dry, but the patient looks very pale to me. What exactly is her blood pressure now?'*
- It is essential to consider what you want to say and do and how you are going to say and do it. Consider your body language and tone of voice so that you do not appear uncooperative or defensive.
- It is important to ensure that you are putting your views across but not imposing them. Negotiation and compromise might be used thus:

  'I think you've given me a full handover but I'm still not happy to take this patient back to the ward now. Would it be alright for me to come back in say, half an hour, or shall I call a more experienced nurse to collect the patient?'

  Rather than: 'No, I'm not taking the patient back to the ward because I don't think she's well enough.'
- If you are inexperienced with regard to collecting patients with a particular piece of equipment or following a specific procedure, for example, you should make this known and seek help from a more experienced practitioner.

Reflection on practice

There will be occasions when the thought of being assertive has caused anxiety and others when the interaction went better than had been anticipated. Reflecting on these events will help to develop effectiveness and confidence on future occasions.

- When considering a similar situation, were you as assertive as you would have liked to have been?
- In such situations what do you think might help or hinder you in fulfilling your objective?
- Are there occasions when you forget the rights of others? Is there a pattern to these occurrences?
- What resources (e.g. self-development books, discussion with your mentor) are there available to help you develop your skills for the future?

NEGOTIATING SKILLS

According to Honey (2001), negotiation involves clarifying what is wanted **(the ideal)** and the minimum that is acceptable for both parties **(the bottom line)**. An example of this is that your mentor meets with you at the end of each shift to discuss your experiences **(ideal)**. The minimum that would be acceptable **(the bottom line)** is that you meet twice a week to discuss your learning experiences, while other qualified nurses contribute to your learning. In the practice situation, referring to the learning outcomes for the placement and being familiar with the opportunities available can help you structure your discussion and negotiate appropriate learning experiences.

Being assertive with your mentor

You are due to have a meeting with your mentor and you are unhappy about some aspects of the relationship and your general experience of being mentored by them.

Some issues raised by this scenario:
- Expressing your needs and wants
- Giving constructive feedback
- Negotiating a desired outcome.

Specific principles

- Being able to work alongside an experienced practitioner is an essential component of an effective practice placement. The Nursing and Midwifery Council (2008b) identifies that a minimum of 40% of the student's clinical experience should be under the direct/indirect supervision of a mentor; this includes an additional hour per week for final year students to be spent with their sign-off mentor. A mentor can act as a role model and enable students to achieve their potential and develop appropriate skills. As you advance through your professional programme, the style of mentorship that will enable you to reach your potential will change. In addition, if you are a midwifery student who is qualified as a registered nurse, there will be skills with which you are already familiar and might therefore need less explanation than someone who has had less exposure to them. You (the mentee) will need to negotiate with your mentors to ensure that they provide effective and appropriate support. If this is not already in place, it would be a good idea to arrange initial, interim and final meetings with your mentor to ensure that your experience continues to meet the outcomes of the placement.
- It can be helpful to have prepared beforehand a written list of issues that you can take to the meeting and which you would like to discuss with your mentor.

- Ideally, the mentorship relationship should be explored and negotiated as near to the beginning of the placement as possible.
- Where discussion of the mentorship relationship does not take place, is one-sided and you are not involved in a collaborative way, or is based on an assumption of your needs, there is likely to be dissatisfaction.
- Preferred styles of mentorship and supervision need to be explored, and strategies for achieving the ideal need to be identified. If there are any obstacles that might affect this, these need to be addressed, e.g. the availability of a co-mentor if your mentor is on night duty or annual/study leave.
- The conversation also needs to include the frequency and location of subsequent meetings to discuss your learning experience.
- While there will always be variation within cultures, where the mentors or mentees come from collectivist cultures (see Ch. 1), there might be a belief that the person seen as the authority figure will offer help without being asked, and a type of dependent relationship may exist (McNamara & Harris 1997). In contrast, the general expectation from an individualistic perspective will be that the mentee will be self-directed and will seek assistance as required. Where mentor and mentee share a similar understanding of how the relationship will operate, there will be a greater sense of satisfaction.

Preparation of self

- Reflect upon what you think is working well and what could be improved.
- Identify what you consider to be your responsibility and that of your mentor, since this might form the basis of the negotiation in your meeting. Using Boud et al's (1985) model of reflection (see Ch. 2) or others such as Gibbs (1989) or Johns (2002), might be helpful.
- You will need to consider what is the bottom line for you, remembering that it needs to be reasonable.
- Consider the nature of the feedback you might be given regarding your performance in the placement thus far. How do you think you might respond to it?
- How are you going to present your concerns? What supporting examples do you have?
- Consulting the link lecturer or your personal tutor before and/or after the meeting might be a supportive strategy.

Environment

- The best time to discuss the mentorship relationship would be during one of the scheduled meetings. The location should be private, where there is less chance of interruptions.
- If meetings have not been arranged, have been cancelled or an urgent situation has arisen, an appropriate time and place need to be chosen to remind the mentor that a discussion is required. It is your responsibility to remind them if necessary.

- As well as alerting the mentor to the fact that you have something you would like to discuss with them, this also facilitates negotiation.

Putting it into practice

- Attract your mentor's attention and state that you would like to discuss your placement, and that you would like to arrange a time to meet. The time between this initial contact and the actual meeting can allow space for both parties to prepare themselves to be constructive.

- Based on your earlier reflective activity, summarize your experience on the ward.

- When giving feedback to the mentor about your experience of the relationship, be clear and specific about your perspective (Seaward 2009). Remember to highlight those areas where the mentor has been helpful, as well as those where things could have been better for you. For example: *'I felt really welcomed when you showed me around the ward on my first day, but now we never seem to be on the same shift and I have not had the chance to work with or speak to you since then.'*

- Avoid generalizations, such as 'everybody's unhappy here', unless you have been asked to speak on behalf of others. Instead, provide constructive feedback that 'owns' your experience by using 'I' statements. For example: *'I realize that this ward is busy and that the staff work very hard, but I'm very unhappy here because no-one seems to have time for me. I'm often left on my own to manage, and I'm not always sure of what I'm doing.'*

- In providing the mentor with this feedback, the skills of empathic understanding (see Ch. 4) and self-disclosure (see Appendix 1) might be used.

- You might choose to tell your mentor how you have been getting on while on the placement, about your experience of mentorship with them and check to see if they have a similar perception to you.

- Alternatively, you can invite your mentor to give feedback about your performance on the ward and how they think the mentorship relationship is progressing.

- When receiving feedback, aim to suspend any judgements until you have heard all of the information, even when you feel anxious about what you might be told; otherwise an ineffective defensive response might result. Honey (2001) suggests that the problem, not the person, should be addressed.

- Additional skills to be employed in the discussion are open and open focused questions, paraphrasing, silence and summarizing. This last skill is particularly valuable during the conversation, since it can help ensure you have heard the key points. It is also useful at the end of a conversation to confirm any actions that have been recommended or agreed.

- Take time to consider your response and agree or disagree as appropriate. It might be helpful to ask for examples if there are areas where you disagree with the feedback. A compromise might be to agree or to disagree on a particular aspect.

- Equally, it is reasonable to ask the mentor for specific examples of your good practice and areas for development, encouraging them to include solutions for areas of concern.
- It is essential that you raise any points that the mentor has not included, but that you consider to be important.
- Identifying a plan of action and a date and time to review the agreed activities would be a good conclusion to this meeting.
- After having attended a meeting, it is beneficial to reflect on what happened in the meeting, your contributions, and the extent to which it met your needs.

Reflection on practice

If you have been in a similar situation:
- How did you feel during the meeting?
- How did your thoughts, feelings and behaviour change throughout the situation?
- To what extent did you achieve any personal aims for attending to the situation or meeting?
- What did you learn about the other person's perspective on the situation?
- How did their perceptions differ from your own? How might you explain this difference?
- What helps you to remain focused during discussions and meetings?
- If you were to have another meeting or discussion (with your mentor), what would you do differently?
- Having considered this scenario, what have you learnt that will help you in this and future placements?

Being an advocate for your patient

While on your placement you are spending the morning observing an interdisciplinary meeting. During the meeting a course of action has been suggested for one of the patients you have been looking after, and you are certain that she would not agree with what is being suggested.

Main issues raised by this scenario:
- Expressing your beliefs and opinions.

Specific principles

- Advocacy is concerned with the promotion and protection of the interests of patients and is a key part of the practitioner's role. When acting as an advocate it is essential to consult the patient or client whenever possible to ensure that their wishes are being represented. There might of course be situations when this is not possible, e.g. where the patient is unconscious. In such a situation, the Nursing and Midwifery Council Code of Conduct should be followed (Nursing and Midwifery Council 2008a).

- At times it might be difficult to be assertive, particularly if you feel that your status in the organization is less valuable than that of the person you wish to address regarding your concern. Lack of assertiveness might also result if you feel that expressing your opinion might not lead to your desired outcome. While this might be the case, expressing your thoughts and opinions signals that you are actively engaged in what is happening. Expressing your opinion might also serve to highlight areas others might not have considered.

- In one's personal life, there might be a preference for responding to situations in a particular way, e.g. passive behaviour; however as a healthcare professional there will be occasions when you need to speak up on behalf of the patient or client. This might involve, e.g. representing their thoughts and feelings while at a meeting.

Preparation of self

- Consider the proposal that is being put forward. How does this relate to what you know about the patient's or client's thoughts and feelings?
- What other information do you need before you express your concern or opinion?
- Are you the best person to raise this concern, or do you need the support of a more experienced practitioner?

Environment

- Is this the appropriate time and place to raise your concern? It might be that only one member of the team needs to be consulted; this could reduce any anxiety that you might have.
- It might be something that could be raised during the ward report rather than at the meeting.
- Is the meeting one where there is free exchange of information?
- Think of an example to support your concern and mentally construct your intervention.
- Keep it clear and concise.

Putting the skills into practice

- Wait for an appropriate pause in the discussion.
- Sit slightly forward and establish eye contact with the person chairing the meeting or the person who last spoke about the area you wish to address. Take two deep breaths and continue to breathe, don't hold your breath and keep both feet firmly on the ground.

- Indicate that you have something to say; pay attention to your body language and ensure that your hands are in a relaxed position.
- Monitor the tone of your voice and speak clearly, fluently and concisely, placing emphasis as appropriate.
- Listen carefully to any comments and feedback.
- Clarify and correct any responses that other members of the team might have made in response to your statement.
- Remember that the team might not agree with you, but you have raised the concern and they can now discuss it with the patient or their family.

Reflection on practice

In situations where you might have been anxious about expressing your opinion, it is useful to spend time exploring your contributions to the situation, so that you can build on the skills that can be used in the future.

- If you have been in a similar situation where you have felt concern, have you been able to say what you wanted to say? If so, make a list of those things that helped you to do so; if not, make a list of those factors which you thought and felt hindered your attempt.
- How do you think your message came across to the other team members? Was it clear and fluent? Reflecting on the nature of any questions that you were asked will provide some information about this.
- When acting as an advocate (this could be for a colleague, a client or a client's relative), to what extent do you think you represented that person's point of view? How did you feel at the time?
- When attending meetings/discussion groups, what, if anything, will you do differently?
- What will you need to consider when giving feedback to the relevant people?

BOUNDARY-MAKING SKILLS

Where we stand in relation to those in our care and our colleagues, is defined by professional boundaries or limits. Boundaries provide containment and physical and psychological safety for practitioners and those with whom they work. Boundaries also ensure that unnecessary intrusions are avoided, i.e. they clarify the extent and limits of professional practice. A sound example of a formal boundary is the law requiring nurses and midwives to meet clearly identified standards of knowledge and skill before they can register with the Nursing and Midwifery Council (2008b). This aims to ensure the safety of the public when using the nursing service (The Nurses', Midwives' and Health Visitors Act 1997). The successful management of boundaries is essential to the making, maintaining and ending of effective professional relationships.

Specific principles

There are a number of principles that apply to the making and maintenance of professional boundaries. Boundaries can be explicit, e.g. the use of formal titles in the workplace instead of first names; or implicit, e.g. the setting-aside of a specific chair for the team leader at meetings without anyone saying this is the case, until an uninformed newcomer sits in it. The more explicit boundaries are, the easier it is for us to be clear of our roles and responsibilities in any given situation, and for colleagues and patients to understand what to expect and where individuals' responsibilities lie. Where boundaries are unclear, confusion can result and the task of care delivery will be lost in any resulting muddle.

Roles

Effective working partnerships are based on mutual respect, which is supported by clear definitions of each other's role and limits to that role – whether a patient, client, family member or practitioner. In order to clarify roles and relationships, it is important to ensure that those with whom we work are aware of who we are and what we are there to do, i.e. the focus of professional practice, at any given time. It is also important that we ourselves and those with whom we are working are clear about these issues, as well as how they fit in with the task of the organization in which we work (Roberts 1994).

Healthcare professionals cross many established social boundaries by virtue of the intimate physical and emotional nature of their work. It is important, therefore, that we understand the **crucial nature of boundaries** to ensure the dignity and comfort of those in our care. Professional colleagues also need to know the purpose of our practice, our expertise and the limits to our skills. We demonstrate our capacity to make and maintain boundaries by our verbal and non-verbal skills, e.g. by introducing ourselves and stating our role, such as staff nurse/midwife, or by wearing a tidy uniform. Boundary-making skills are closely allied to assertiveness skills, because stating and demonstrating limits, need unambiguous verbal and non-verbal statements of who we are and what our roles and limits are. This means we need to use assertive verbal and non-verbal skills (see above).

Boundary-making skills

Sully (2003) identified a number of skills involved in making and maintaining boundaries. Self-awareness of feelings, thoughts and actions as well as the limits to our own responsibilities and abilities is required, as well as skills in negotiating explicit working contracts, including the limits to the situation or relationship, e.g. clarifying the task at hand, others' responsibilities, time and working environment.

Assertive language and non-verbal skills are required, e.g. saying 'no' clearly (Clark 2003, Ch. 4) and having an assertive as opposed to aggressive or submissive posture; agreeing and keeping to time limits, such as stating the time and duration of an interview with a client or relatives and keeping to this decision. The observation of process skills is important, e.g. raising what you observe is happening or has happened in a particular incident to keep task-focused or to clarify what has actually been happening. Active listening and immediacy skills (addressing the here-and-now) are required, as is empathy (seeing the situation from the other person's point of view), as opposed to identification with the others and the situation. This means 'being with' someone in distress (Benner 2001: 50) but not allowing any intense feelings of your own, evoked by their situation, to confuse your thoughts and actions.

Problem-solving and decision-making skills are required, as are skills in leaving the issue behind, e.g. by choosing to do so, changing clothes, not discussing the issues outside a given time limit, or informally, by changing activities then or later. The effective use of professional supervision, where exploration of practice and constructive feedback and support can be sought and given, is also important. Box 6.2 provides examples of some common boundaries.

Box 6.2 Examples of boundaries

- **Hierarchy** enables the practitioner to refer to those more senior such as the Patch Manager for guidance, or indeed to make a final decision; and to act as a support or guide to someone junior, such as the staff nurse to the student

- **Uniform** identifies each practitioner's role and status, clarifying what can and cannot be reasonably expected of the practitioner. This effectively limits and contains the individual's practice and helps ensure the recipient can identify the practitioner's social and professional role

- **Codes of conduct** clarify what is and is not acceptable practice. They should safeguard the public and support practitioners by stating clearly their responsibilities

- **Terms of address:** these set boundaries, e.g. by ensuring formality in a situation that could be embarrassing. An example of this is the consultant gynaecologist who addresses his patients, with whom he was on first-name terms, as 'madam' during a vaginal examination

- **Contracts of employment:** these agreements stipulate the responsibilities of employers as well as employees, thus providing a framework for practice and due reward and the processes to follow when the agreement is violated

- **Time:** stating the specific amount of time you have available to work with patients ensures that they know when the appointment with you will end. This can provide a sense of security, particularly for people facing frightening procedures

- **Space** by its nature contains and/or limits activity. For example, it is necessary to have enough space around a patient's bed to employ a hoist

- **Environment:** certain activities can only occur in certain places such as operating theatres.

Wearing your own clothes on placement

You are going on a community visit with the health visitor. You are aware that you need to be appropriately dressed, but are unsure of the dress code.

Some issues raised by this scenario:

- The need to consider the nature of the work you will be doing in the placement
- The importance of considering the impact that your dress might have on the people with whom you will be working – both colleagues and clients
- The variety of tasks you might be undertaking and how this might influence your choice of clothing
- In the community you are likely to encounter situations in clients' homes that are unfamiliar to you.

Specific principles

- It is important to consider not only what image you want to present, but also the cultural diversity of the community. It is important to wear clothes that will not cause offence to people of different ages, genders and cultures.
- It is advisable to clarify with your supervisor or the placement manager what dress code is expected.
- The nature of the work you will be doing each day, e.g. visiting patients or clients in their homes, assisting in a Child Health Clinic, or working in a Day Unit, will inform you about what clothes are appropriate for the tasks you are likely to undertake.
- If you are likely to be working in a variety of different and possibly unfamiliar environments, it is advisable to wear clothes that are modest, comfortable and inexpensive but professional.

Preparation of self

- What are your feelings, thoughts and actions in relation to this situation?
- What working contract have you negotiated with the health visitor; e.g. place, date and time of meeting? What are you expected to do during the visit?
- How assertive can you be in order to clarify what is expected of you?
- Do you know how long the visit is likely to take? What will you do if the visit extends over the time agreed, or if the health visitor has to alter the arrangements?
- Clothes need to be appropriate for the situation and task. What sort of clothes are you considering wearing? A useful *aide mémoire* is: **LHSLT**. Appropriate clothes are: not too low, not too high, not too short, not too long, not too tight.

Environment

- When working in the community, it is not always possible to have much control over the environment, as much of the practice goes on in private homes. However, it is crucial that nurses and midwives can state clearly their needs for as suitable an environment as possible for carrying out their duties in environments where they have no formal control; e.g. ensuring they have the correct equipment for weighing a baby or moving and handling.
- What do you know about the community in which you will be visiting, its general health, social mix and customs? Have you clarified whether or not you are visiting a home or community where there is a strict dress code such as keeping your upper arms covered?

Putting the skills into practice

- Contact the health visitor by telephone or face-to-face. This personal contact supports the establishment of a working rapport. Clarify the purpose of the visit, where it is likely to happen and ask about the dress code.
- Ensure you know when and where you are to meet and whether you are likely to be walking or using some form of transport.
- Ask the health visitor whether what you intend to wear is appropriate in that community.
- Dress neatly with clean clothes and shoes. Ensure the length of your trousers or skirts is formal and thus demonstrates professionalism. Do not wear clothes with political slogans or risqué jokes.

Reflection on practice

Reflect on a situation from your nursing or midwifery experience when you have needed to clarify a boundary about dress at work.

- How did you feel when you decided to take the initiative and clarify the boundary of appropriate dress?
- How did the person you asked respond to your taking this initiative?
- What effect did their response have on your discussions about appropriate dress?
- How much influence did different cultural expectations have on your choice of dress?
- How will what you have learnt from this situation affect the development of your communication skills?

Using humour to make a polite refusal

A client who is being discharged asks you to come out for a drink that evening to celebrate 'newfound freedom'.

Some issues raised by this scenario:

- The relationship between nurse and patient, or midwife and woman, is one of unequal power.
- Patients and pregnant women or those who have newly delivered their babies are vulnerable. A consequence of this might be that they seek ways to overcome the power imbalance by trying to set up social situations where they can be in control. This might be precipitated by a change in their health status or situation, such as when they are being discharged and therefore feel more able to assert their autonomy.
- The client might be seeking a relationship with you that is social and/ or possibly sexual. Accepting this offer would be inappropriate as your relationship is formal and based on the understanding (stated or not) that you will not abuse the power you have had entrusted to you.
- There is also the issue of your vulnerability, e.g. to unfounded allegations of accepting social benefits or encouraging sexual advances, or to having your privacy violated by being waited for outside the hospital or health centre and followed home.

Preparation of self

- What are your feelings, thoughts and actions in relation to this situation?
- If you are likely to feel uncomfortable, embarrassed or offended, how may this affect your ability to respond with humour?
- Think of light-hearted terms that could be used in response to the patient's or woman's own terminology, e.g. the use of the word 'freedom' could elicit a response using the word 'escaping'.
- How much time have you spent working with this client? How well do you know them? Would you both enjoy a laugh together?
- What are your responsibilities as a practitioner to maintain professional boundaries? How do you regard this in relation to socializing with patients, women and carers?
- How assertive can you be in order to draw the professional boundaries here, while using a light-hearted response?

Environment

- Where is this situation likely to occur? It is probably in the ward or Outpatients Department if you work in a hospital, but it could be a rehabilitation centre or a specialist clinic, or mother and baby unit.
- Where is it best to address this crossed boundary? How much control over the environment do you have?
- While it is essential to be respectful, in the interests of a sound therapeutic relationship and the maintenance of your client's dignity, you also need to consider your potential vulnerability to having your response to this

invitation misconstrued. Avoid dealing with it where you cannot be seen and/or heard by other members of staff.

- It is preferable to deal with this situation in a public place where you can *both* be seen, e.g. with the bed or cubicle curtains drawn open.

Putting the skills into practice

- Adopt an assertive stance – not too close in proximity (this might be interpreted as aggressive or collusive) but upright and relaxed.
- Look directly at the client, bearing in mind possible cultural and gender differences in understanding non-verbal cues.
- Draw the boundary by stating a clear but polite refusal, offering a light-hearted response.
- Use humour, but recognize the client's need to celebrate this event.
- Link your response to what the patient has said by using the assertive skill of restating or paraphrasing their words. This demonstrates empathy in that you have heard how they have experienced their situation, e.g. this client sounded as if they found a stay in hospital or the unit particularly restrictive.
- Avoid put-downs and rude comments. You could say: '*So you're escaping at last! You must be looking forward to going home. A drink is a good way to celebrate with your friends and family. I'm afraid I can't join you, but have a great time!*'

Reflection on practice

Think of a situation from your experience when you have had to draw a boundary with a client using humour.

- What was difficult about drawing the boundary with the client?
- How did your feelings influence the way you responded?
- How did the client react to your response?
- How much influence did different cultural expectations have on your response?
- How will what you have learnt from this incident affect the development of your communication skills?

References

Atkinson, T., Claxton, G. (Eds.), 2000. The Intuitive Practitioner: On the Value of Not Always Knowing What One is Doing. Open University Press, Buckingham.

Benner, P.E., 2001. From Novice to Expert: Excellence and Power in Clinical Nursing Practice. Commemorative edn. Addison-Wesley, Menlo Park.

Berne, E., 1975. What Do You Say After You Say Hello? Corgi, London.

Bond, M., 1986. Stress and Self-Awareness. Heinemann, London.

Boud, D., Keogh, K., Walker, D., 1985. Reflection: Turning Experience into Practice. Kogan Page, London.

Clark, C.C., 2003. Holistic Assertiveness Skills for Nurses. Springer, New York.

Dickson, A., 1982. A Woman in Your Own Right. Quartet, London.

Gibbs, G., 1989. Learning by Doing: A Guide to Teaching and Learning Methods. Oxford Polytechnic, Oxford.

Harris, T., 2004. I'm OK – You're OK. Avon Books, London.

Honey, P., 2001. Improve Your People Skills. IPM, Wimbledon.

Johns, C., 2002. Guided Reflection: Advancing Practice. Blackwell Science, London.

Kim, M.S., 1995. Toward a theory of conversational constraints. In: Wiseman, R. (Ed.), Intercultural Communication Theory. Sage, London, pp. 148–169.

McFall, M., Winnett, R., Bordewick, M., 1982. Non-verbal components in the communication of assertiveness. Behav. Modif. 6, 121–140.

McNamara, D., Harris, R. (Eds.), 1997. Overseas Students in Higher Education. Routledge, London.

Nursing and Midwifery Council, 2008a. Code of Professional Conduct. Nursing and Midwifery Council, London. Online. Available at: www.nmc-uk.org/aArticle.aspx?ArticleID=3056 (accessed 13 March 2009).

Nursing and Midwifery Council, 2008b. Standards to Support Learning and Assessment in Practice. Nursing and Midwifery Council, London.

Nurses', Midwives' and Health Visitors' Act, 1997. Online. Available at: www.opsi.gov.uk/ACTS/acts1997/ukpga_19970024_en_1 (accessed 19 July 2009).

Oetzel, J., 1995. Intercultural small groups: an effective decision-making theory. In: Wiseman, R. (Ed.), Intercultural Communication Theory. Sage, London, pp. 247–270.

Paul, N., 1985. The Right To Be You. Chartwell-Bratt, Bromley.

Rakos, R., 1991. Assertive Behaviour: Theory, Research and Training. Routledge, London.

Reed, H., 2003. Criteria for safe discharge of patients from the recovery room. Nurs. Times 99 (38), 22–24.

Roberts, V.Z., 1994. The organization of work. In: Obholzer, A., Roberts, V.Z. (Eds.), The Unconscious at Work: Individual and Organizational Stress in the Human Services. Routledge, London, pp. 28–38.

Seaward, B., 2009. Managing Stress: Principles and Strategies for Health and Well-Being, 6th edn. Jones Bartlett, London.

Singelis, T., 1994. Bridging the gap between culture and communication. In: Bouvry, A., Van de Vijer, F., Boski, P. (Eds.), Journeys into Cross-cultural Psychology. Swets & Zeitlinger, Amsterdam.

Stewart, I., 2007. Transactional Analysis Counselling in Action, 3rd edn. Sage, London.

Sully, P.A., 2003. Communication in adult nursing. In: Brooker, C., Nicol, M. (Eds.), Adult Nursing: The Practice of Caring. Elsevier, Edinburgh.

Witte, K., Morrison, K., 1995. Intercultural and cross-cultural health communication: understanding people and motivating healthy behaviours. In: Wiseman, R. (Ed.), Intercultural Communication Theory. Sage, London.

Further reading
Dryden, W., Constantinou, D., 2004. Assertiveness Step by Step. Sheldon Press, London.

Hartley, M., 2006. The Assertiveness Handbook. Sheldon Press, London.

Hayes, J., 2002. Interpersonal Skills at Work. Routledge, Hove.

Hoban, V., 2003. How to … handle a handover. Nurs. Times 99 (9), 54–55.

Nicol, M., Bavin, C., Bedford-Turner, S., Cronin, P., Rawlings-Anderson, K., 2008. Essential Nursing Skills, 3rd edn. Mosby, Edinburgh.

7

Communicating where barriers exist

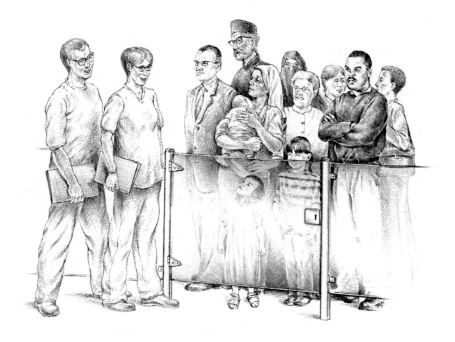

INTRODUCTION

As health care practitioners we communicate in a wide variety of environments, on multiple occasions with an infinite variety of people, often using equipment such as the telephone, facsimile machine, e-mail and visual aids such as cue cards. The focus of this chapter is the development of skills to communicate effectively across barriers. There are situations where this may be difficult and misperceptions and misunderstandings may result.

This chapter aims to address some of the situations where effective communication requires specific consideration. The chapter is divided into two sections, the first addressing telephone skills and the second outlining other situations where effective communication might be difficult. These include the use of appropriate language; assisting people who are deaf or hard of hearing; assisting people who are blind or partially sighted; assisting people who have dementia; using cue cards effectively and the importance of being aware of the resources available for interpretation.

TELEPHONE SKILLS

Speaking on the telephone is, for most people, an everyday occurrence. It is a means of both social and professional communication. There are, however, certain conventions that are acceptable in social discourse on the telephone that would be inappropriate in professional circumstances, e.g. how we greet the caller when we answer the telephone. Although we cannot see each other while speaking on the telephone, strong impressions about one another and the organization, can be transmitted. It is important therefore to develop skills in using the telephone in order to convey a courteous and efficient manner and develop appropriate professional relationships with callers.

Throughout the working day, there are a number of experiences that remain in your preconscious and/or unconscious but will have an effect on your practice and communication. Furthermore, in some instances callers will try to elicit information which they know they are not party to, from staff over the telephone.

Answering the telephone when you are busy

The ward is very busy and one member of staff is off sick. You are busy with a patient or client but notice that the telephone has been ringing for some time. Having excused yourself from the person in your care, you answer the telephone.

This scenario explores how these experiences might influence your telephone manner and how any negative experiences might be prevented.

Principles

- The telephone does not provide the visual information that is used to complement communication that occurs during face-to-face conversation. This lack of visual information and contact means that hearing needs to be finely attuned.

- If you are having or have had a difficult day, your tiredness or irritability might be inadvertently evident in your tone or the words you use.

- It is important to signal the opening and closing of the conversation. The opening of the conversation must include personal identity and the location.

- Listening skills need to be more finely attuned to particular aspects of communication, e.g. the caller's tone of voice, any pauses in the conversation, what is said/not said or what is implied.

- Careful consideration needs to be given to how any questions are worded.

- Always ensure that the caller has a legitimate reason for obtaining/is authorized to be given information.

- Clear coherent speech, with clarification sought at regular intervals, is essential.

- If the caller is to be left while further information is obtained, he or she should be informed of the forthcoming break in communication and the reason for this. The 'secrecy' button should then be used while the caller is awaiting your return to prevent other conversations being overheard.

  Note: See chapter 5 on safeguarding patient/client confidentiality.

Preparation of self

- You need to be aware of how you feel about being short-staffed as well as being interrupted while you were giving care.

- Taking a deep breath, clearing your mind and smiling might help you dissipate any anger or frustration you might have. Standing firmly on the ground or sitting rather than shifting from one foot to another might help you remain calm and focused. It's not the caller's fault that you are having a difficult day!

- It would also be helpful if you consider that the caller might also be anxious or frustrated about the nature of the call they are making and the difficulties they might have had getting through to the ward (Farrell 1996).

Environment

- What else is going on in the ward that might affect the quality of your telephone conversation?

- Who else can hear the conversation you are about to have? It might be appropriate to transfer the caller to a quieter and more private location.

Putting the skills into practice

- Make sure that you leave your patient or client safe and comfortable before leaving to answer the phone.
- Identify the ward, your status and your name, in a clear and unhurried manner. If the caller has not already stated what they want, ask how you can help.
- Apologize for the fact that the caller has been kept waiting.
- If the caller starts the conversation before you have had the opportunity to do any of the above, you will need to listen to what they have to say and give the information at an appropriate point.
- It is important not to become defensive if the caller complains about how long they have had to wait to get through to the ward. Telling the caller that you are busy might at times be appropriate. However, this is not an intervention that addresses the caller's concerns; in fact it might exacerbate them, particularly if they take this to mean that the staff are too busy to look after their relative.
- Adjust your tone accordingly to reflect the nature of the conversation.
- Deal with the caller's enquiry with confidence and repeat the apology in your parting statement.

Reflection on practice

Think of a situation from your experience where you have answered the telephone when busy.

- How would you ensure that the person in your care was safe and comfortable before leaving to answer the phone?
- When in similar situations on the telephone, do you consider that you have presented a calm and reassuring manner?
- If you have been calm in such situations and able to reassure the caller, how did you manage to achieve this?
- If, on reflection, you felt hurried and less understanding of the caller's needs than you could be, what would you need to do differently if a similar situation arose again?
- Were you able to provide the information that the caller required? If not, what other resources were available to you?
- Having ended the conversation, was there anything else you wished you had said or done? How are you going to increase the likelihood of remembering these aspects in the future?
- If you have to leave a patient or client to attend to another issue, consider how you might respond if they seem to be annoyed or feel inconvenienced (see also Ch. 8, "Dealing with embarrassing situations").

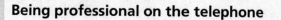

Being professional on the telephone

A caller asks you about the condition of a relative. You do not know who the patient is.

The importance of establishing and maintaining trust and confidence over the telephone is addressed in this scenario.

Preparation of self

- Consider how the caller might be feeling.
- Identify the name of the unit and introduce yourself.
- Think of a statement that will be reassuring and lets the caller know that even although you do not know the patient, you are still concerned and wish to help them.
- Take a deep breath, relax and smile, this will help your voice sound warmer and reflect interest and enthusiasm.

Environment

- What else is going on in the ward that might affect the quality of your telephone conversation?
- Who else can hear the conversation you are about to have? It might be appropriate to transfer the caller to a quieter and more private location.

Putting the skills into practice

- Identify the ward, your status and your name in a clear and unhurried manner. If the caller has not already stated what they want, ask how you can help them.
- Inform the caller that you will go and speak to the person in charge rather than saying, 'I don't know who that is' or 'I've never heard of that patient'. A more appropriate response would be to say that you are *not familiar with that particular patient*.
- Before leaving to seek this information from other staff members, inform the caller that you are going to get further information and apply the 'secrecy' button.
- On returning to the caller, let them know who you are transferring them to before passing the receiver to the staff member.

Reflection on practice

- When in situations where you have been distracted while giving care, you will need to consider whether your attitude and manner led the caller to feel confident in you as a professional practitioner. If so, how did you achieve this? If not, what could you do differently?

- In similar situations where you have to pass information on to other people, what information do they need in order to help a third party efficiently?
- Having put the receiver down or handed the caller over to someone else, have there been times when you wished you had said or done something differently? By reflecting on such a situation you can continue to develop and improve your skills and confidence.

Maintaining confidentiality on the telephone

A caller enquires about a relative and asks you what sort of illnesses are treated on the ward.

Some issues raised by this scenario:
- Maintaining patient confidentiality when an anxious relative is requesting information
- Strategies for maintaining professional competence and reassuring relatives.

Putting the skills into practice

- Identify the ward, your status and your name in a clear and unhurried manner. If the caller has not already stated what they want, ask how you can help them.
- Permission should always be obtained from the individuals in your care before you pass on any information concerning their presence on your unit or their details/condition to enquirers. It is crucial that any inadvertent direct or indirect disclosure of the presence of a patient or woman being in your care or on your ward, is always avoided. This issue is crucial when a person is fleeing from their partner because of domestic violence, e.g. a pregnant or newly delivered woman is at increased risk of being killed by her current or former partner (see Richards 2003 and Ch. 5).
- Ascertain exactly who the caller is and let them know that you will see if the patient is awake and able to speak with them. If the patient does not wish to or is unable to speak with the caller, take a message, repeating it to the patient in order to ensure that you convey their wishes to the caller.
- If the caller asks for more information relating to the nature of the patient's condition or nature of the ward speciality, politely decline to disclose this unless there is a previous agreement with the patient about who can have information about their condition (see above).
- It might be appropriate to refer to an external authority, such as the hospital or professional policy by saying that it is hospital policy not to give such information. However, internalized professional values relating to respecting privacy and maintaining confidentiality, along with the ability to demonstrate these with ease, are signs of an expert practitioner.
- If the patient consents for information to be given, it is important that you consider the words that you are going to use, since you might not

know the circumstances and condition of the caller. It is generally useful to establish when the caller last saw their relative. If the patient's condition has deteriorated, you might say something like: *'There is some concern about her/his condition now.'* If this is the case, consider whether you need to ask someone with more experience to take the call.

Reflection on practice

- When speaking to concerned relatives over the telephone, to what extent have you been able to address the caller's enquiry efficiently?

- Have there been any aspects of patient confidentiality that you found difficult to maintain over the telephone or face-to-face with a relative?

- What additional information or resources will help you if dealing with a similar call in future?

- If you were the last person to speak with the caller, having put the receiver down, was there anything else you wished you had said or done? How are you going to increase the likelihood of remembering these aspects in the future?

Taking test results over the telephone

A member of staff from the laboratory rings with a patient's blood test results.

When conveyed over the telephone, information can be distorted, leading to numerical information being misinterpreted and resulting in patient safety being compromised. This scenario identifies a procedure to enhance accurate recording of information given over the telephone.

Putting the skills into practice

- Identify the ward, your status and your name in a clear and unhurried manner. If the caller has not already stated what they want, ask how you can help them.

- Since you might need to call back to clarify a piece of information, it is essential that you ascertain the name of the person to whom you are speaking.

- Ask the caller to wait while you get something to record the information on. There might be a designated book for this or the information might go directly into the patient's records.

- Write each result down and check spelling and figures as you go.

- Once the results have been given, repeat these to the caller before the call ends.

- Inform the person in charge that the results have arrived. The doctor might also need to be informed.

- If you are a student, your signature will need to be countersigned by a qualified practitioner when you have entered the results in the appropriate place.

Reflection on practice

- When taking results over the telephone, what will you need to do to ensure that you have accurately received all the appropriate information?
- What additional information and equipment might you need to enable you to record the information appropriately?
- How are you going to ensure that you pass on this information accurately to the appropriate person or people?
- Were there results or information that you did not understand? Aim to find out what they mean and their significance to the care you are providing and the overall treatment plan.

COMMUNICATING WHERE BARRIERS EXIST

One of the greatest challenges in nursing and midwifery practice is to be able to communicate effectively with those in our care and their families when barriers to communication exist. When caring for patients and clients who have communication difficulties, it is important that we consider how we might demonstrate the core conditions of helping and building effective therapeutic relationships with those in our care. In order to do so, we need to bear in mind how patients and clients might be feeling and thinking and how this might affect their behaviour and that of their families.

There are many potential barriers to communication that nurses and midwives will regularly need to deal with, e.g. deafness, language differences and speech impairment following a stroke. In midwifery, particularly on the labour ward, relationships sometimes have to be established in a quick and trusting manner in order to facilitate the optimum outcome for mother and baby. Consider what barriers to effective communication you have experienced in practice and what you did to overcome them.

Imagine you are in a foreign country where you do not speak the language. You suddenly have terrible abdominal pain and need help. What might you be thinking? How might you feel? How will you be able to explain your needs to people who come to your aid? People who cannot speak English, and those who are blind, deaf or disabled by learning difficulties, brain injury or illness causing thought and memory impairment – or confusion because of shock, or dementia associated with ageing – are also likely to face these thoughts and feelings when they are distressed or ill and need help.

Factors influencing communication

Whaley & Wong (1991) identified a number of factors that influence communication:

- Perceptions (how we see ourselves, others and the situations we are in)

- Values (which underpin our ethical decisions, thoughts about them and behaviour)
- Development (our age and life stage affect how we perceive and experience situations)
- Personal space (proximity and how we use the space around us have an impact on how we are perceived and how we feel)
- Emotions (can be very powerful and have significant consequences for effective communication)
- Sociocultural background (see Ch. 1 for the implications of this)
- Knowledge (this gives us a framework of reference and can be used as a means of power and control, as in expert power, described by Grasha (1995: 358, after Raven 1992)
- Roles and relationships (social status and relationships, both formal and informal, influence communication)
- Environment (this is addressed throughout the text as significant in all interactions between people).

The model of communication that underpins the approach of this book (see Ch. 1) highlights the significance of our personal history, social history and our history in society. These issues are likely to become more obvious when barriers exist and we are trying to communicate effectively across them. These histories affect both our conscious and unconscious processes and might reflect unhelpful attitudes that, in turn, reflect the prejudices of society.

Principles

In order to communicate effectively where barriers exist, we need to consider a number of principles.

Therapeutic relationship

The provision of the core conditions of warmth and respect, empathetic understanding and openness and genuineness (Rogers 1957) are as crucial here as in any other therapeutic relationship. When people have difficulties in communicating, offering these conditions will help them to feel safe and cared for, even although they might have problems expressing their needs. The ways in which we demonstrate these core conditions are likely to be subtly different from how we would do so when we are communicating where there are no barriers. An example of this could be that we might give more eye contact when talking to someone who is deaf.

Language issues

The use of dialect or specific expressions varies across different parts of the country but also among age groups, social backgrounds and people with disabilities. It is important to bear this in mind when we are talking to people where there are communication difficulties, as they may use language that is unfamiliar to us or that means something different from what is expected by us. Not being aware of this possibility can add to the risks of misunderstanding and confusion. Regional and foreign accents can impede verbal communication and mutual understanding. In the area of your practice it is important to consider whether your way of speaking and use of non-verbal cues could be a barrier to effective communication. For example, a Yorkshire accent may be unintelligible to an elderly person born and brought up in the East End of London. This is a similar situation for first generation migrants, regardless of whether they are the carers or the people receiving the care.

Working with people when barriers to communication exist frequently takes more time than when there are no difficulties. It is therefore important to make enough time available to listen to your clients' and patients' needs and explain the care they are receiving. This skill is an important way to demonstrate respect and empathy. Take care to avoid using inappropriate terms of endearment or controlling language, e.g. 'dear', 'lovey', 'good boy'. This demonstrates disrespect and is discourteous. It is important always to check your understanding of the patients' needs as well as clarifying their understanding of what you have communicated, with them (see Chs 5 and 10).

Being honest about not understanding and thus asking clients to repeat what they have said is an essential skill (Brearley & Birchley 1994). It demonstrates respect and concern for the client and can reassure them that you are making a genuine effort to understand. However, it is important to do this without displaying signs of irritation. Sometimes we might have particular anxieties about disabilities or situations where communication is likely to be difficult. If we are aware of our own anxieties in these circumstances, we are more likely to be sensitive and patient, particularly when we are under pressure.

Cultural issues

All societies have norms and values about people's roles and status. It is important to bear in mind the cultures from which those in our care come as well as our own culture and that in which we work. Discriminatory attitudes such as ageism (Le May 1998, Scrutton 1999) do occur and may influence how those we care for perceive us and how we perceive them. Self-awareness is particularly important when we communicate where barriers exist because unconscious prejudices may hinder the successful building of therapeutic relationships.

Our assumptions about people's ability to communicate can be influenced by a variety of factors such as the situation or our previous experience, with the consequence that we make inappropriate assessments of how extensive the hindrances to communication are. An example here is that in some cultures a woman may not say anything in front of her husband, as it is important that she defers to him in public. Practitioners might then assume that she cannot speak English, which is not necessarily the case. Being aware of, and using formal interpreting services in practice is essential. Confidentiality can easily be broken by inappropriate use of family members or other patients as interpreters. This can result in patients not disclosing their needs or indeed these not being explained, with the result that appropriate care is not offered.

Deafness and partial sight

Never assume that everyone who comes for healthcare can see and/or hear. If a patient has not responded to their name, always check that they have seen and/or heard you. This also applies in hospitals and residential homes when meals and drinks are brought. Always let the patients know you have brought them a meal. Social definitions of disability can be prescribed by those without the disability, e.g. use of the term 'hearing loss' sounds like a medical definition with an emphasis on the **lack** of hearing ability, whereas deaf people prefer the positive description 'deaf' as this describes them as they **are**, not as lacking the ability to hear.

Dementia and cognitive difficulties

Where people have chronic communication difficulties resulting from illness like dementia, it is important to have an understanding of how their illness has affected their speech and interaction with others. How we respond to others is not only about how well we know them, but also about the social context and physical environment as well as the nature of our relationship with them (see Ch. 1). If illness impairs memory and/or the ability to think about who one is and thus one's sense of self as well as how you want to express your needs, communication becomes very difficult (see Ch. 4).

Aids to communication

In the UK, the Disability Discrimination Act 2005 requires all public organizations to:

- Promote equality of opportunity between disabled persons and other persons
- Eliminate discrimination that is unlawful under the Act.

This duty means that people with disabilities must be offered services according to their needs, even if it means offering more facilities to them than to people without disabilities (Disability Rights Commission 2005: 2.13). It is therefore important to recognize that communication aids are central to sound care delivery and should be available in all healthcare settings. Likewise the provision of sign language interpreters for deaf people is a responsibility of the public authorities providing the services (see Disability Discrimination Act 2005).

Aids to communication such as cue or picture cards, pen and paper are essential equipment in any healthcare setting. Sign language used by deaf people has its own social conventions, vernacular and dialect. British Sign Language has now been recognized by the UK government as an official language. It can be helpful for practitioners to learn some sign language in order to develop professional relationships with clients and colleagues.

USING APPROPRIATE LANGUAGE

Colloquial language

Mr Richard Laycock is a 90-year-old man who is admitted to your ward for treatment of a chest infection. He is breathless and feeling unwell. You are allocated to do his nursing assessment. He greets you briefly but with a smile and says: *'My, but I'm crook, nurse!'*

Some issues raised by this scenario:

- Mr Laycock is considerably older than the staff. His language is likely therefore to be of his generation.
- The use of the word 'crook' (meaning unwell) might be confusing to others. It does not mean he is a dishonest person, i.e. a crook!
- His breathlessness means that talking is likely to be exhausting.

Specific principles

- It is important to consider Mr Laycock's age. His use of language is likely to be of his generation and therefore different from yours.
- Respect is demonstrated by clarifying how he prefers to be addressed (see Ch. 3), and by avoiding the use of inappropriate terms of endearment such as 'darling'. This latter can be perceived as condescending.
- Communication is a two-way process, so if you do not understand any terms he uses, it is important to ask for clarification.
- Use language that is unambiguous and does not require long explanations. Avoid jargon (Le May 1998). For example: *'For how long have you been breathless?'* requires a short answer like: *'Three days.'* This ensures Mr Laycock can give you a specific answer without a long explanation.
- Allow time for Mr Laycock to express his needs, which should be actively sought even although you are trying to limit the demands on his strength.
- Avoid controlling language such as leading questions like: 'You aren't bothered too much by the oxygen mask, are you, Mr Laycock?' This does little to enhance his trust in you (Le May 1998) and does not demonstrate respect.

Preparation of self

- Think about how you feel about Mr Laycock's condition. Have you cared for an older adult with similar health problems and communication difficulties?
- Consider carefully what you want to ask Mr Laycock in the assessment; his breathlessness will make long explanations difficult and tiring.
- Think about how you are feeling. You might feel apprehensive about asking too much of a patient in obvious distress.

- Consider what sort of information you need from Mr Laycock in order to do an accurate assessment of his needs. Decide what information can wait until he is a bit better, so you don't demand too much from him at this first meeting. What information can be gained from other sources, e.g. the medical notes or an accompanying relative?
- What is the best way for you to gain this information? Closed questions require short answers. These are more appropriate for Mr Laycock, as talking is likely to be strenuous and stressful for him.
- How will you open, conduct and close the interview?
- Think about what you have noticed about Mr Laycock's demeanour. Is he cheerful when you are with him but subdued and struggling to relax when he is not talking to anyone? How will this influence the language and questions you choose and the tone of your voice?

Environment

- Ideally this should be private, out of earshot and quiet so Mr Laycock does not have to raise his voice to be heard. This can be difficult to attain on an open ward, but pulling the curtains partially or completely around the bed can help to muffle sound and offers privacy.
  Note: He might find the enclosing nature of the curtains adds to his respiratory distress as he might experience the closed curtains as confining and restricting the flow of air.
- Consider where you will position yourself in relation to Mr Laycock. You need to be close enough for him to see you and for you to hear him, but take care not to assume a proximity that might seem discourteous or intrusive. It is important not to crowd him as he is breathless and might experience this as suffocating.

Putting the skills into practice

- What you observe about Mr Laycock will guide you as to how to open the interview so you can avoid putting unnecessary demands on him for lengthy explanations. This would also apply to a patient in pain.
- Approach his bed quietly as he has respiratory distress. Consider where you will position yourself. A chair near his bed is probably best so he does not feel crowded.
- Make your greeting and introduction short but friendly. A short social interaction such as: 'It is nice to meet you, Mr Laycock' is appropriate here but social chit-chat extends the interaction and could add to his discomfort.
- When you begin your assessment it is important to explain your reasons for the questions you are asking and that you will try to phrase them so that he only needs to give short answers.
- Clarify with him any terms he might use, like 'crook', by asking: '"Crook" isn't a term I fully understand. Does it mean that you feel really unwell?'

Reflection on practice

Think about a situation from your nursing experience when you cared for someone with respiratory distress or in pain.

- What were your feelings while you were working with the patient? How do you think they influenced the way you spoke and the language you chose?
- How successful were you in keeping your language clear and straightforward? What questions seemed most effective?
- How successful were you in helping to avoid the patient having to give long-winded explanations?
- What would you like to have done differently? What observations of yourself and your patient's responses prompted you to consider these changes?
- What feedback did you give the nursing team in order that they understand your patient's communication needs? How, when and where did you give it? What did you document in the care plan?

Using culturally sensitive language

Joshua is a young man of 17 years old. He is getting out of bed for the first time since he fractured his tibia and fibula in a motorcycle collision. You are helping him to sit comfortably in a chair beside his bed. Once he is safely in the chair you ask him how he feels. He replies: 'It's cool to be out of bed! *My leg is OK, but I feel as if my arse belongs to someone else!*'

Some issues raised by this scenario:
- Confusion might arise from the use of the word 'cool', i.e. it might be interpreted as his feeling cold now he is out of bed.
- The use of the term 'arse' might be offensive to other patients within earshot and indeed some nurses might find it vulgar and not respectful towards them.

Specific principles

- It is important to consider Joshua's age and developmental stage. He is in late adolescence and probably still vulnerable to feelings of insecurity and thus uncertainty about how to behave appropriately. These feelings might mean that he behaves with bravado or he might appear withdrawn or moody, i.e. he might create barriers to effective communication.
- Careful consideration needs to be given to how Joshua might be feeling as a developing young man suddenly dependent on others to do intimate things for him, at a time when he is gaining independence and becoming increasingly adult. This is particularly significant if the nurses are not

much older than he is. Consequently, Joshua might adopt behaviour that aims perhaps, to shock or irritate in order to assert his independence. Your response needs to take into account his age and his feelings about how this situation affects his sexual and self-image (Hoff et al 2009, Price & Gwin 2007).

- It is important that we are aware of our response, why we are making it and what our feelings are. We might be the parents of adolescent children and want to respond to him as we would to our own children. However, if we respond to him in this way we might say something insensitive. This awareness will help us avoid negative responses, which are likely to create our own barriers to effective communication (see Ch. 1).

- As a teenager Joshua uses language that is part of his subculture. It is important therefore that what he actually means is clarified. When he says 'cool', does this mean he is cold, or is he really pleased to be more independent and out of bed?

- Use age-appropriate language. Joshua is old enough to understand formal language for anatomy and physiology, but avoid using long technical terms, which practitioners sometimes resort to when they are embarrassed or ill at ease.

- In order to demonstrate genuineness it is important to avoid using language with which we do not feel comfortable and which we would not use ourselves.

- Using terms like 'arse' might be something you feel comfortable with, but it can offend others. It is important to consider what image you are presenting when you use language that might offend or shock – maybe not Joshua himself, but those around him. This language might be appropriate when talking to Joshua but might not be if the patient were from a different background or age group.

- It is also important to remember that if we use inappropriate language, we can cross professional boundaries and those in our care might feel less sure of how to relate to us.

Preparation of self

- Think about how you feel about Joshua's situation. How do you feel about a young man being so badly injured and subsequently dependent?

- What reactions did you have to his language use? What language would you use instead without seeming to be critical of Joshua's preferred terminology?

- Consider carefully how you are going to clarify exactly what Joshua means when he says his 'arse doesn't feel as if it belongs to him'. What sort of information do you need from Joshua to help him feel more comfortable?

- What language will you use to describe his discomfort while he is sitting?

- Think about what you have noticed about Joshua's demeanour. Is he trying to cover up pain by bravado? How will you deal with this?

Environment

- Joshua is in a chair beside his bed and in view of the rest of the ward. Other patients might be watching to see how you respond to him and his reaction. It might be the first time since his admission that he has been in a position where he can have more relaxed interaction with ambulant patients and visitors.

- Consider your proximity to Joshua before you address his concerns about his 'arse'. Positioning yourself too closely to him might feel embarrassing or intrusive.

- If you need to attend to his discomfort, remember to close the curtains so that you do not expose him and cause him embarrassment.

Putting the skills into practice

- Respond to Joshua in a friendly and open way.

- Stand near him and perhaps to one side and try to keep your eyes level with his. This is likely to entail crouching down to his level or sitting on a stool or chair. Avoid stooping over him as he might feel this is intimidating.

- Ask him to explain exactly what he means when he mentions his discomfort. You might say: *'That sounds very uncomfortable, Joshua. What exactly is the sensation that you have now you are sitting in a chair and which part of you feels as if it doesn't belong to you?'*

- Clarify with him any terms he might use like 'cool' if you are unfamiliar with his vernacular. You might say with a smile: *'The word "cool" can have several meanings. What exactly did you mean when you said it was "cool" to be out of bed?'*

- Draw the curtains round and help Joshua to get comfortable. If you feel he was making some sort of sexual innuendo out of bravado or embarrassment it is wise to ask someone to help you so he is not alone with you.

- It is important to engage his cooperation in repositioning him so it is a collaborative exercise as opposed to you 'doing something' to him. Be clear about how you want to help him reposition himself.

- Be matter-of-fact if you need to alter his clothes or uncover him in any way that might risk embarrassing him. You might say something like: *'I'm going to need to lift your pyjama top. Perhaps you'd like to hold the blanket to keep yourself covered.'*

- Consider what you will document in his care plan.

Reflection on practice

Think of a situation from your practice when you have cared for someone who was particularly sensitive to intimate care and the dependence it brought. Consider their use of colloquial language and how this might have been a means of covering their embarrassment.

- When you asked about the patient's comfort how did you feel about their response? You might have felt as if you hadn't 'got it quite right'. How do you think your feelings influenced the way you spoke to the patient and the language you chose? If you were embarrassed by the patient's language, how did you deal with that?

- If you had to ask the patient what they meant by their colloquialism ('cool' in Joshua's case), how did they respond?

- How successful were you in keeping your language clear and straightforward? What instructions seemed most effective in helping to get your patient's cooperation during the care process?

- What, if anything, would you like to have done differently? What observations of yourself and your patient's responses prompted you to consider these changes to your practice?

ASSISTING PEOPLE WHO ARE DEAF OR HARD OF HEARING

(With grateful acknowledgements to Julie Hornsby (2009, 2004) and Sharon Lee (2004), sign language interpreters.)

If someone is deaf or hard of hearing they have a disability that is not necessarily obvious when we first encounter them. This can put them at a disadvantage if we do not assess their needs effectively. In a birthing environment, the woman is likely to be concerned and anxious not just for herself, but also for her baby. She may feel that options offered may be limited because of her difficulties. As we are likely to care for people who are deaf or hard of hearing, it is essential that we develop our skills of communicating with them effectively and sensitively in order to meet their nursing and midwifery needs appropriately.

In the UK, most service providers – such as Primary Care Trusts – will have service level agreements to provide sign language interpreters. These practitioners can be contacted through local authorities or an agency such as the Royal National Institute for the Deaf. It is also possible to have a deaf intermediary present (Casson-Webb & Wood 2009), particularly in situations that might entail legal reports, which can help the deaf person and the intermediary develop a rapport as the intermediary might have met the deaf person before the actual interview.

Giving directions to a person who is deaf or hard of hearing

You are standing in the busy entrance to the hospital waiting to meet a colleague when a middle-aged woman who looks very distracted comes up to you and asks for directions to the Outpatients Department. You notice that she has a rather flat intonation to her voice, the words are slurred and she seems to stare at you as she speaks. You have to ask her to repeat her question. When you begin to explain she says: 'I'm sorry but I don't hear you very well. Please would you repeat that?' You then notice that she has a hearing aid.

Some issues raised by this scenario:

- The woman's manner might at first seem anxious and her intense gaze perhaps a little rude. When people have difficulty hearing and the situation is unfamiliar it can exacerbate their feelings of anxiety.
- The environment is noisy and this is likely to make it more difficult for a person with hearing loss to understand you.

Specific principles

- Often people are tempted to raise their voices when someone is hard of hearing. This is not helpful as it can distort their lip patterns and make it more difficult for the person to lip read.
- As there are many causes of deafness and different forms of hearing loss, this underlines the importance of assessing individual needs and adjusting your communication strategy accordingly. For example, you might need a sign language interpreter and/or to use cue cards.
- It is important to assess the client's ability to hear in that environment and adjust your response accordingly.
- Best practice is always to carry a pen and paper while at work in case you are asked to help someone who is deaf.
- Drawing pictures and enabling the deaf person to do so too, will aid effective communication.
- Help the person to understand by pointing to the equipment or apparatus to be used and make appropriate gestures/movements, e.g. positioning yourself where you would like the person to be and pointing to the couch or chair.
- If it is an unfamiliar situation for you, prepare yourself by practising how you will convey what is required of the person in that situation and how you will structure your communication.
- People who have no speech can sometimes lip read, so even if you do not know sign language, always try and face a deaf or hard-of-hearing person when you are speaking to them.
- Never touch people with hearing loss before they have seen you. They probably will not have heard you approaching and this can give them an unpleasant surprise. It is also disrespectful.
- Wherever possible, it is best practice to use a registered interpreter for deaf people rather than an enthusiastic amateur. Family members should be used with caution to protect privacy and confidentiality and ensure accurate interpreting.
- Always consider your employer's policies and practices about booking and using interpreters for deaf people. It is important to bear in mind that more notice is often required than is needed for interpreters for spoken languages.

Preparation of self

- Consider what your priorities are in this situation. You are meeting a colleague, but a hospital client needs your help. How might you help the client but not miss your colleague?

- Think about your feelings. You might be embarrassed that you cannot fully understand what the client is saying, particularly as deaf people can have indistinct speech; or you might be anxious that you will miss your colleague. Acknowledging your feelings and putting them to one side helps to ensure that they do not interfere with the way in which you communicate verbally and non-verbally with the woman.

- Decide on how you will invite the client to move to somewhere more suitable in which to talk and think about how best to give her clear and logical directions to the department requested. Consider the structure of your sentences as well as the language you will use. Always use short words and sentences.

- Consider whether you need to draw her a map, or find a clear hospital plan to show her.

Environment

- This environment is noisy and distracting. Therefore, it is important to suggest moving to a quieter place so the client can see and hear you better.

- If it is not possible to find a quiet area or corridor, or it is inappropriate to go outside, make a quieter space by moving aside to a wall or into a quiet corner.

Putting the skills into practice

- Be friendly and smile as this demonstrates that you are willing to help.

- Suggest that you move to one side and indicate this with your hands if necessary, demonstrating the need for a quieter, less busy place in which to talk.

- Be aware of how you are feeling so that you can use your feelings to help you communicate effectively rather than allowing them to interfere with your practice.

- Encourage a collaborative relationship by explaining to your client that you need to be within view of the main entrance, so she understands if you are unable to find somewhere quieter, well away from the entrance.

- Telling her your name and asking her for hers can help encourage a collaborative relationship. It is important to wear your name badge and to draw it to her attention.

- Position yourself so that the client can see her surroundings as well as seeing your face clearly. Ensure that you do not hem her in if you have to stand to one side in the entrance area. **Do not stand in front of a door or window,**

as the light behind you will obscure your lip patterns. Position the client in front of the door or window instead.

- It is important to talk slowly while facing the woman so she has the optimum opportunity to lip read (Quill 1995, Craddock 1991). Keep your voice well-modulated and at a normal pitch. Raising your voice is not necessary and, depending on the type of deafness, can make it more difficult for the client to understand.

- If it is difficult to understand what you are being asked, it is important to request that the person repeats the question, possibly using 'different words' (Brearley & Birchley 1994: 62), or ask her to write her request.

- Explain the directions logically, using clear simple sentences and beginning from where you both are now standing. Complicated directions can be confusing. Indicate by gesture the signs visible around you and the direction she should take. If necessary, draw her a map if you have a pen and paper with you, or show her the way.

- You might ask her if she knows familiar landmarks or places in the hospital on the way to the Outpatients Department. This helps to put your directions into context.

- When you have finished, ask her if she is now clear about how to find the Outpatients Department or whether she would like to repeat any of the information.

- When you part, it can be reassuring to say you were pleased you could help.

Reflection on practice

Think about a situation when you had to communicate with someone who was deaf or hard of hearing.

- Some deaf people have visual impairments too (e.g. Usher's syndrome). Had you considered that the person you were seeing might have this or other disabilities too? Were you able to check their records beforehand, to ensure you were well-informed about their situations/diagnoses and specific needs? If not, how did you deal with the situation?

- What did you feel when you first met the person you were going to help? You might have felt anxious that you would not communicate effectively, or irritated because the communication was taking much longer than you felt you had time for. You might have felt embarrassed because it took you a while to realize the person was deaf. You might also have felt uncomfortable if their speech was difficult to understand.

- How successful were you at putting your feelings to one side so you could engage fully with the needs of the person? What helped and/or hindered this process?

- How did your thoughts and feelings influence the way you spoke and the language you chose?

- How successful were you in keeping your language clear and the sentences straightforward? How did the person respond?

- What would you like to have done differently? What observations of yourself and the client's responses prompted you to consider these changes to your practice when communicating with people who are deaf or hard of hearing?
- Consider what training needs you might have. It is always useful to learn a few words of sign language such as 'deaf', 'hello', 'good-bye', 'please' and 'thank you'. How do you think you would benefit from classes in British Sign Language?

ASSISTING PEOPLE WHO ARE BLIND OR PARTIALLY SIGHTED

(With grateful acknowledgements to Eric Gallacher, retired physiotherapist, London, July 2009.)

People who are blind or partially sighted have their own particular communication needs. It is helpful to develop a wide vocabulary so we are able to describe the care we give succinctly. Non-verbal cues are felt rather than seen, therefore it is important we are sensitive about how we use touch and language in order to communicate effectively with people with these disabilities.

Escorting a blind person

You are a student nurse on placement in a large general practice and are working with the practice nurse in the treatment room. She asks you to go to the waiting area to collect Mrs Josephs, a 50-year-old woman who is blind, and bring her to the treatment room to have sutures removed from her arm.

Some issues raised by this scenario:

- The waiting area is likely to be noisy. Because the background noise might muffle the sound of your footsteps and she cannot see you, it is important to consider how to approach Mrs Josephs without giving her an unpleasant surprise.
- Consider where you will position yourself before you speak to her, and when and how you will touch her.

Specific principles

- Always introduce yourself to the client and state your role, before offering a service to the blind client.
- People who are blind or partially sighted often have more enhanced and sensitive hearing. Therefore speak initially with a gently modulated and relatively quiet voice. A raised voice that is heard suddenly can be startling. It is important not to start speaking to blind people when you are behind them. This too can be disconcerting.

- Blind people need to be told when meals or drinks have been served, what they consist of and whether they would like assistance with their food such as help to cut the meat. Using the face of the clock to describe the relative position of things, such as: *'Potatoes are at 9 o'clock and meat at 12 o'clock'*, might help.

- Touch is a very important form of communication for blind people. They use it to understand their surroundings as well as to read and write. Consequently, they can be very sensitive to how they are touched by others.

- Touching blind people before speaking to them is intrusive, can also be an unpleasant surprise and does not demonstrate respect or empathy for their situation. Therefore always speak before you touch them.

- Often people are tempted to take control and lead the blind person to their destination. Instead you should regard yourself as the agent for enabling the blind person to get there safely. It is important to consider how best to help Mrs Josephs walk to the treatment room and ask her how she prefers to be escorted. Generally blind people prefer to hold your elbow rather than you hold theirs. This allows them a sense of control.

- Blind people can memorize the layout of familiar places. Assess how well Mrs Josephs knows the geography of the surgery and the position of furniture and equipment in the treatment room.

- Clearly describe any hazards ahead, for example a step up or down, a door that opens towards you.

Preparation of self

- Think about your feelings. You might be unsure of how you will approach Mrs Josephs, particularly as you are aware that blind people can have very sensitive hearing. Acknowledging your feelings and putting them to one side again helps to ensure that they do not interfere with the way in which you communicate verbally and non-verbally with her.

- Think of strategies to overcome any blocking feelings such as shyness. For example you might think about a brief story in the news that you might want to mention to Mrs Josephs as a way of breaking the ice. The weather is also a good topic. After all, she does not know you either and might feel anxious about who will escort her and how efficient they will be.

- Familiarize yourself with the layout of the route you intend to take and the position of furniture and equipment in the treatment room. You need to know exactly where you are going if you are to escort Mrs Josephs smoothly and confidently to where she needs to be. Note any dangerous obstacles and decide how you will circumvent them. If possible, move any obstacles before you collect Mrs Josephs.

- Remember never to touch her before speaking to her.

- Decide on the language you will use to explain that you have come to escort her to the treatment room. Choose words that will enhance partnership as opposed to language that could be received as controlling or 'taking charge'. For example: *'I have come to help you to the treatment room. How would you prefer me to escort you?'*

- Describe any features on the way, e.g. whether the doors open towards you or away from you and whether steps go up or down.

Environment

- As the waiting area is likely to be busy and noisy, consider how you will ensure as far as possible that this does not interfere with how you make yourself known to Mrs Josephs. This could be by getting in close proximity to her when you talk to her and explaining that there are a number of people moving about. Speak clearly in well-modulated tones and avoid trying to shout above the noise.
- Notice the position of the furniture in the waiting area and on the route to the treatment room. Notice too where there are doors or the likelihood of people coming out from adjoining rooms, or any other hazards.

Putting the skills into practice

- Approach the person you understand to be Mrs Josephs and position yourself in front but somewhat to the side of where she is sitting.
- Do not touch her before you have spoken to her and introduced yourself. Use a relatively quiet tone to introduce yourself and clarify that the patient is Mrs Josephs. As part of your introduction you might like to shake her hand as this is a socially acceptable form of touch and lays the foundations for touching her in order to escort her.
- Explain who you are and that you have come to escort her to the treatment room to see the practice nurse for her appointment.
- If Mrs Josephs seems ill at ease or you feel shy, it can help to make a short social remark like: *'Sometimes when it is very busy in here like today, it feels as if the work won't ever get done in time.'* If she has been waiting past her appointment time, you could demonstrate respect and empathy by apologizing for keeping her waiting.
- Assess how well Mrs Josephs knows the geography of the surgery by asking whether she has been there before and how familiar she is with its layout. Clarify any parts of the layout she doesn't know or doesn't remember.
- Promote partnership by asking how she finds it best to be guided. Ask whether she would prefer to hold your elbow or for you to hold her, which side she would prefer you to stand and whether she would find it helpful if you explain the route as you go along. Blind people usually prefer to hold your elbow, as this positions you slightly in front of them so they can feel any change in your position. This is the same technique used with a guide dog.
- Guide Mrs Josephs in her preferred manner. Touch should be firm and reassuring, not hard and rigid. Remember Mrs Josephs has sutures in her arm, so avoid contact with the arm that has the wound.

- Use touch to accompany your verbal explanations and descriptions of your route. Depending on how Mrs Josephs prefers to be guided, she can feel in which direction you are going by feeling your elbow which indicates, e.g. the direction you will turn a corner or if you slow down before an obstacle like a swing door.

- Escort her to the treatment room using clear descriptions of any obstacles or features on your route such as the height of steps, the position of swing doors or other features.

- If you need to take a route that is not familiar to her, explain your reasons for this.

- When you arrive, help Mrs Josephs to the chair or couch and assist her to get comfortable, explaining exactly where the chair or couch is in relation to her. For example, you might say: 'The couch is diagonally ahead of you, about two feet to your right', and escort her to it. Allow her time to feel it for position and structure so she can control how she settles herself on to it. It can be helpful to put the client's hand on the arm or back of the chair or side of the couch. State where the head and the foot of the couch are, so they can gauge where to move.

- If the practice nurse has not already greeted Mrs Josephs, introduce her.

- Negotiate with Mrs Josephs and the practice nurse about whether you will be needed during the suture removal. After the treatment has been completed and Mrs Josephs' wound is comfortable, escort her back to the waiting area.

- If she needs to sit down for a while before going home or on to work, ensure she is comfortable and check that she has a reliable means of getting to her next destination: if not, offer to arrange this for her.

- Take your leave of Mrs Josephs. You might like to shake her hand as you say goodbye.

Reflection on practice

Consider a situation from your practice when you were asked to escort a blind or partially sighted person.

- What was it like to be with someone who could not see you clearly, if at all? Consider how this affected the ways in which you interacted with them.

- How did you feel? You might have felt apprehensive about the person bumping into things.

- How successful were you at putting your feelings to one side so you could relate respectfully and empathetically to the person? What helped and/or hindered this process?

- How did your thoughts and feelings influence the way you spoke and the language you chose?

- How did the person respond when you introduced yourself? How did you negotiate the best way in which to escort the person? How successful were you in giving clear descriptions of your route? What descriptions were most effective in ensuring your passage was smooth?

- How did touch influence the way you and the person interacted? Consider their verbal and non-verbal responses to your verbal and non-verbal directions.
- How successful do you think you were in helping the person to feel comfortable and safe during this process? What indications were there for you to come to these conclusions?
- What, if anything, would you like to have done differently? What prompted you to consider these changes to your verbal and non-verbal communication with blind people?

ASSISTING PEOPLE WHO HAVE DEMENTIA

People who have dementia demonstrate a change, i.e. a deterioration, of their functioning compared with their previous abilities. These changes involve 'all or most functions associated with intellect and memory' (Jolley 2005: 22). The consequences include changes to their 'personality' (Jolley 2005: 22) the manifestations of which vary from person to person. They have progressive difficulties with memory, their sense of who they are, and thus their sense of themselves and their concentration and ability to speak. One of their communication problems is that they find following and being involved in conversations increasingly difficult.

Note: In the UK, it is possible to install in the client's home a small radio-operated system called *Just Checking* (Department of Health 2009a) to monitor how your client is managing their everyday activities. Family members, carers and professional teams are able, through internet access, to assess and monitor their loved ones'/clients' conditions, abilities and safety by reading the reports relayed on line.
Some issues raised by this scenario:

Assisting a person who has dementia

Mr Groves is a white Caucasian man aged 76. He is living in a residential home where you have been working for the last 2 months. You have been asked to work with Mr Groves as the qualified nurse who usually leads the team caring for him is on annual leave. Sometimes you have worked with that team and understand that Mr Groves asserts his independence whenever he can. He does not however remember you, as his memory and concentration spans are very limited. You are also aware that if he is not given a choice on personal issues such as where to sit in the day room, or the order in which he dresses himself, he becomes distressed and resists any attempts to assist him. It is lunch time. He is able to eat with the other residents and you invite him to come to the table. He looks at you uncomprehendingly and says, 'Just got up.'

The meal is due to be served in a few minutes and you know that Mr Groves dislikes food he describes as 'cold'. You would like him to come to the table but are reluctant to hurry him.

- Mr Groves is clearly unsure of the time.
- You are not someone he is familiar with and so is less likely to remember who you are.

Specific principles

(See Ch. 3; Bayles & Tomoeda 2007 and Harris 2005.)

- It is important wherever possible to support people with dementia in their daily choices, rather than impose decisions upon them. Nursing care should 'promote dignity by nurturing and supporting the older person's self-respect and self-worth' (Nursing and Midwifery Council 2008).
- Recognize that people need time to understand what is required of them as well as to carry out activities of daily living. People with dementia often need more time than you might foresee, to carry out a task such as dressing or walking to a dining table.
- Use language that is courteous and clear and reflects their status as an adult. It is important to avoid 'elderspeak', i.e. language that demonstrates a sense of the speaker's superiority and that infantilizes the older person. Examples are described by Williams et al (2009: 12) as 'using simplistic vocabulary and grammar, shortened sentences, slowed speech, elevated pitch and volume, and inappropriately intimate terms of endearment' such as 'darling' and 'sweetheart'. This manner is disrespectful and uncaring.
- Adults with dementia are more likely to resist care interventions and requests to behave in a particular way such as coming to the table, if 'elderspeak' is used (Williams et al 2009).
- It is important to acknowledge the experiences and feelings of people with dementia. Practitioners who ignore their clients' feelings or insist that their perspectives are irrelevant or 'wrong' and consequently disallow them the expression of their needs and choices, can contribute to loss of self-esteem, and an increase in depression, withdrawal and dependent behaviour (Ryan et al 1986).
- Among the communication difficulties people with dementia have are mispronouncing or using inappropriate words, difficulty in remembering conversations and taking turns in conversations (see Harris 2005 for a detailed discussion).
- When speaking to people with dementia it is important to remember that they have impaired memory and find long and complicated sentences difficult to comprehend.
- Help the person to understand by offering more than one means of explaining, such as using pictures or writing and allowing the person to read the instruction to support what you are saying.
- Use straightforward and simple sentences, without excessive detail, and straightforward vocabulary.

- Remember that the person with dementia can lose their understanding if there are numerous people talking together. This situation can lead to their becoming agitated. Avoid overwhelming the person with more than one or two people in the interaction.

- Use a pleasant and well-modulated voice and a calm, measured rate of speech. Fast speech can be difficult to hear, as well as being confusing for those having difficulty comprehending. Remember too, that many older adults have hearing difficulties and this can complicate the person with dementia's ability to understand.

- If your client does not understand, repeat what you have said using different vocabulary.

- Talk about the present when requesting a client's involvement in their care or explaining the situation.

- Repeat the names of people and things, e.g. '*Mr Groves, your chair is placed the way you like to have your chair placed*' instead of 'Your chair is ready the way you like to have it'. This sentence doesn't use the pronoun 'it', as this can be confusing (Bayles & Tomoeda 2007).

- Offering people with dementia choices in their daily activities (Department of Health 2009b) is central to respectful, holistic and person-centred service provision and is likely to reduce their 'resistiveness' (Williams et al 2009).

Preparation of self

- Think about your experiences so far with people with dementia. You might have found that you are particularly sensitive to their needs and have been effective in enabling them to maintain their independence in their activities of daily living. Recognizing your skills as well as aspects of working with people with dementia that have caused you anxiety, can help you to address how to use your abilities to overcome any concerns you might have in making a relationship with Mr Groves.

- Think of strategies to help Mr Groves to understand that lunch is due to be served. Construct a straightforward sentence in your mind that you will use to invite him to come to the table. You might know from working with him before and from his records that he likes to be escorted to the table. You can therefore offer to walk with him or help him if he needs assistance with his mobility.

- Consider how you will gain his attention and keep him in the present. It is important to acknowledge his experience of being confused about the time. One way of helping him understand that it is later in the day than he thinks, is to observe that he is dressed and where he is, i.e. in the day room not in his bedroom. Consider how you will position yourself in order to gain his attention but without intruding in his personal space unnecessarily.

Environment

- The residential home might be noisy. Try and talk to Mr Groves away from the distractions of talk or the noise of cutlery.
- Ensure his place at the table is ready for him so that he can sit down and is less likely to be distracted from the present.

Putting the skills into practice

- Approach Mr Groves so that he can see you coming towards him. Position yourself so you are not leaning over him – this posture can feel domineering – or standing too far away so he cannot see that you intend to have a conversation with him.
- Stand where the light is to the side or in front of you – not behind you which makes your face difficult for Mr Groves to see.
- Greet him by name. Speak to him in straightforward, simple sentences. Say that lunch is ready and you have come to help him to the table.
- As he seems confused about the time, gently clarify the time, e.g. it is 12.30, and show him the clock or your watch. Invite him to come with you to the dining room.
- If he is reluctant to agree, *'avoid confrontation'* (Harris 2005: 125, italics added). Gently suggest that you understand that he seems to be feeling uncertain as to whether it is lunch time and offer him an alternative such as having his lunch brought to him.
- It might help too if you explain what is on the menu, without giving him a long list!
- Walk with him to the table if he decides he wants to eat there. Before helping him to sit down, offer to help him, rather than assume he wants your intervention. These strategies offer Mr Groves choices. Help him with his chair, if this is necessary. If he is able to sit down without assistance, allow him to go at his own pace.
- Again, offer him the same choice of food when he is at the table. If he changes his mind about what he wants to eat, respond empathetically and offer him the alternatives.

Reflection on practice

Think about a situation from your practice when you have worked with someone with dementia.

- How did the person relate to others? Were they irritable, withdrawn or 'compliant', offering no response to you when you offered care, conversation or tried to engage them in an activity of daily living?
- What did you think were the reasons for their behaviour and levels of involvement in their care and/or environment? If they were withdrawn or 'compliant', were there other indications such as a sense of their having 'given up' in trying to have some autonomy or choice in their daily existences?

- If they were resistive and unwilling for you to help them with their activities of daily living, communal activities such as singing or in therapies such as reminiscence therapy, how did staff, other residents and visitors speak to them? Was 'elderspeak' part of the culture of the residential home where they lived, or had lived in the past?

- What strategies did you use to involve the person helping them to have choices such as in what they wore or ate?

- How effective were you in establishing a rapport with the person?

- If you felt strong emotions such as fear that this might happen to you, anxiety in that you seemed to be achieving little to ensure the person received appropriate care without being denied the dignity every person is entitled to, how did you deal with them so they did not interfere with your capacity to offer gentle and considerate care?

- What verbal and non-verbal interventions did you use to help attract and maintain the person's attention? How effective were they?

USING CUE CARDS AND PICTURE BOARDS

Cue cards and picture boards are cards or boards showing symbols and/or pictures which staff and those in their care can use to communicate with one another. They can be used to indicate experiences such as feeling pain, particular situations, patients' needs and treatment prescribed. Cue cards and picture boards are available, or can be developed, for individual clinical areas. They are useful for people who do not speak English or those who have cognitive difficulties in either expressing themselves verbally, as with people who have aphasia, or for those who cannot read or have limited language skills. They can be particularly useful with patients suffering from aphasia.

Chapey & Hallowell (2001: 3) define aphasia as an acquired communication disorder caused by brain damage, characterized by an impairment of language modalities: speaking, listening, reading and writing. They state that aphasia is not caused by mental health disorders, sensory or general intellectual deficits. Aphasia has a profound impact on the individual's sense of identity (Parr et al 2003a,b). People become aphasic usually following a head injury, stroke or some other event. They are likely to grieve for their lost abilities to relate to others through speech and to enjoy the creativity and versatility of verbal language and humour (Boazman 2003). They face a significant time of transition and might need specialist emotional help with their sense of loss and their change of self-identity.

There are significant social and relationship impacts for adults who develop aphasia. It is therefore important that practitioners take into account their clients' feelings about the impact their aphasia has on their intimate and social relationships, as well as on the wider issues of their lives such as their employment and leisure activities (Lubinski 2001).

Note: Aphasia and dysphasia mean difficulties in expressing oneself through speech. In some earlier texts, the terms 'aphasia' and 'dysphasia' are used interchangeably (Norman & Redfern 1997).

Assisting a person with aphasia

You are a third-year student nurse on placement in a Rehabilitation Unit for older adults. Ms Frank is a 60-year-old former head teacher who has had a stroke. She likes to have a wash every morning in the bathroom and you have been asked to help her. She has left-sided hemiplegia but is able to mobilize. Her speech has been compromised and she has difficulty speaking, but she can understand what you say. She is an independent woman who tries hard to manage by herself.

Some issues raised by this scenario:

- The difficulties encountered when communicating with someone who understands but cannot speak
- The frustration felt by patients with aphasia.

Specific principles

- When we are working with people with aphasia it is important to remember that intense feelings, that might be exacerbated when they struggle to communicate, can influence their abilities to speak.
- They can also experience a loss of control; that in turn can be intensified if they are also having to face physical disabilities such as hemiplegia following a stroke and/or loss of mobility.
- People with aphasia usually need more time to communicate than those without this disability. Practitioners therefore need to be patient and not hurry the individual.
- It is important also to speak in a more measured pace, rather than the quicker speech delivery common in Western communities.
- Because of their reduced ability to process language quickly, people with aphasia might lose the capacity to be humorous or to engage in casual banter. It is important for practitioners to be aware of this so as not to assume that the person with aphasia has no understanding of a gentle joke. Similarly, it is important not to use humour inappropriately as this could be, however inadvertently, insensitive and possibly unkind.
- Just as the causes of aphasia differ, so people who are aphasic do not have the same manifestations of the problem. Careful assessment of their needs is crucially important.

- Listening carefully to understand the message underneath what might seem to be bizarre language takes patience and skill. Self-awareness is very important. Anxiety that you will not understand or will not be able to give the patient or client enough time to express themselves can interfere with your capacity to understand (Brearley & Birchley 1994).

- Giving time to those in our care is one way of demonstrating respect, as it can help them feel valued. This is an important emotion for most people, but for those who face a devastating life change through the loss of the ability to communicate effectively and thus to have control of their lives, that someone has taken the time to engage with them and listen, can be a very important experience to them.

- Accompanying disabilities such as hemiplegia might mean that they are also unable to use gestures or writing to express themselves. Therefore practitioners need to recognize that while for some people drawing pictures or writing one or two words might be an appropriate way to express themselves, for others this is not possible (see Clarke & Clarke 2003).

- Aids to communication such as cue cards and picture boards, pens and small dry-wipe writing boards are therefore essential tools.

- Although it is helpful to be advised about their needs and preferences and what certain sounds or gestures mean, by people who know the aphasic person well, it is important to try and enable the person to communicate their needs without requiring the constant presence and intervention of someone else (Brearley & Birchley 1994). The constant involvement of others can feel disempowering for the client and might be a breach of their confidentiality.

- Avoid language that is condescending, e.g. calling Ms Frank by endearments rather than by her name; or controlling language such as only using closed questions and not allowing opportunities for alternatives to be chosen or indicated on the cards.

- Always try to remember that although you feel frustrated and despair at not being able to communicate effectively and thus meet the needs of the aphasic person as sensitively as you would like, they are likely to feel a deep sense of frustration and despair on their side too.

Note: For a detailed list of options for communication interventions for people with aphasia (see Appendix 4).

Preparation of self

- Think about your feelings. You might be feeling uncomfortable about helping such an independent resident to bath herself, particularly as she was a head teacher and as such, a person with authority. You might feel embarrassed that you cannot understand what she says, particularly as her speech is bizarre at times; or you might be anxious that you will not meet your own standards of patience and respect. Acknowledging your feelings and putting them to one side helps to ensure that they do not interfere with the way you relate to Ms Frank and how you communicate with her verbally and non-verbally.

- Check her nursing notes to see how Ms Frank likes to be helped to mobilize, whether she prefers a bath or shower and what toiletries she uses. If nothing is recorded, ask members of the nursing team if they are aware of any of these preferences. This will enable you to clarify with Ms Frank exactly how she would like you to help her.

- Consider consulting a speech and language therapist for guidance about communicating more effectively with Ms Frank.

- Try to relax and take your time. Rushing to communicate with and help Ms Frank to the bathroom will not demonstrate respect for her and her condition. Your anxiety can be easily picked up by Ms Frank and might add to her own. This added stress might make her speech more erratic and incomprehensible, to the distress of you both.

- Decide on how you will explain to her that you will be helping her to the bathroom to wash. Think about what order the cue cards should be in so that Ms Frank can find them readily and explain her needs and answer any questions.

- Be sure that you have all the equipment you need to help her to the bathroom such as a walking frame. Ensure that you know where to find her towels, clothes and toiletries.

Environment

- Consider the layout of the Rehabilitation Unit. Is Ms Frank's bed in a general ward or in a side room? How private is this if it means you are going to take some time to explain, using cue cards, that you will be helping to bath her?

- Is there a suitable surface on which to display the cards, e.g. bed table or tray?

- How much room is there for you to manoeuvre around her bed so you can assist her to the bathroom? What route will you take? Is the bathroom free and what equipment (e.g. hoist or chair) might you need?

Putting the skills into practice

- Think about how you are feeling. Try to be as relaxed as possible, so that any anxieties you might have about communicating with Ms Frank do not influence your interactions with her.

- Considering how Ms Frank feels, having had a responsible and authoritative position, and now being unable and physically dependent on others, will enable you to empathize with her in her changed circumstances.

- Approach Ms Frank in a friendly manner and, if she does not already know you, introduce yourself by name.

- Promoting partnership with her in her care demonstrates respect for her autonomy. You might say: *'I will be working with you this morning, Ms Frank. Please let me know how you would prefer to be helped in the bathroom.'*

- Ensure you have the cue cards to aid communication with Ms Frank. Put the cue cards where both you and she can see and use them. You might need to help her select them so using her bed table might be the best space on which to spread them out.

- Check that you have all the equipment you need ready to help her to, from and in the bathroom.

- Allow sufficient time to help Ms Frank, as communicating with her will take longer than it would with someone without a speech impediment. She is also likely to need a lot of time to wash.

- Explain that you are going to help her to wash. Although this is the time she usually prefers to go to the bathroom, check that she would indeed like to wash now and if not, when she would like to do so.

- Position yourself so that Ms Frank can see you and both of you can see and use the cards. Avoid standing over her as she might experience this as intimidating or feel that you are in a hurry. You might say: *'I have brought these cue cards to use to help us in case we don't understand each other.'*

- Use straightforward closed or open focused questions that need short answers to clarify how she prefers to be helped to mobilize, what toiletries she uses, whether she prefers a shower or a bath, and how she would like to be helped in the bathroom.

- Help her to use the cards to identify her needs and preferences. You might need to move them around and offer different ones if Ms Frank is having trouble answering your questions or stating her needs. If you are asking her for her preference, hold up the cards that show the options, e.g. one for the bath and one for the shower. Take the cards with you to the bathroom so they are available if you need them.

- Demonstrate respect and empathy by ensuring your non-verbal cues are relaxed so you do not seem in a hurry, anxious or impatient.

Reflection on practice

Think about a situation from your experience where you have had to communicate using cue cards or a picture board, in order to give care to a patient or client.

- How successful were you at communicating effectively with the patient and engaging them as a partner in their care? What observations did you make that led you to these conclusions?

- How did you feel during the episode of care? You might have felt anxious, frustrated or out of your depth; if so, how did you deal with your feelings?

- What particular interventions helped you to work with the patient or client while using the cue cards? What, if anything, would you have done differently?

- How did touch influence the way you and the person in your care interacted? Consider their verbal and non-verbal responses to your verbal and non-verbal cues.

- How successful do you think you were in helping them to feel respected, private and safe during the care episode? What indications were there for you to come to these conclusions?

- What would you like to have done differently? What observations of yourself and your patient's or client's responses prompted you to consider these changes to your practice of communicating, using these tools?

WORKING WITH INTERPRETERS

The UK has a multicultural and multilingual heritage, with a population that reflects richly diverse cultures and beliefs from around the world. Not everyone, however, speaks the official language of the country in which they live, in this case English.

Working with a language interpreter

You are working in a surgical ward. One of your patients, Mrs Begum, aged 45, has been admitted for a laparoscopic investigation for chronic abdominal pain. She will be in hospital overnight and has no pain at present. She speaks Bengali but no English. She is accompanied by her 19-year-old son who speaks fluent English. He offers to interpret for his mother.

Some issues raised by this scenario:

- How is it possible to make a truly collaborative therapeutic relationship with Mrs Begum if she cannot speak English and you cannot speak her mother tongue of Bengali?

- Mrs Begum's son has offered to interpret for his mother but if he does his mother will be denied the right to confidentiality in her healthcare (Nursing and Midwifery Council 2008). It is not always possible to find a professional interpreter when most needed, so if Mrs Begum gives her consent, her son could interpret for you both. However, this situation is far from ideal as it can be very embarrassing for them, e.g. when discussing topics such as menstruation, contraception and conditions relating to sexual activity such as sexually transmitted diseases.

- Practitioners **must** take great care that they do not assume consent or put Mrs Begum in a compromising situation, such as not asking to see her alone to give her the opportunity to communicate in private. She might speak some English but cultural norms might require that she defers to the men in her family in public. It is very important therefore *never* to assume that because in public someone defers to their elders or the men in the family, that they do not speak English.

Specific principles

- Practitioners need to be aware that there are 'ethical, legal and professional implications' (Ledger 2002: 773) in the manner in which they communicate with those in their care who cannot speak English. When family members or members in the patients' communities are asked to interpret, not only are the patients' rights to confidentiality violated, but interpreters are also put in an invidious position of keeping confidences or perhaps not having the technical language to interpret accurately. Professional and personal boundaries are crossed inappropriately when this occurs (see Ch. 6).

- In these situations there is also the risk that, for reasons of modesty, culture or at worst, power and control, interpretations are edited or incorrect. This is particularly important when considering vulnerable families, especially those at risk of violence from the wider community or those where there is intimate partner violence, elder and/or child abuse.

- As stated above, *never* assume, if a client does not speak for themselves while their spouse or another family member answers for them, that they cannot speak and/or understand English. It might be that they feel intimidated when family members are present.

- Consider asking relatives to write common phrases in Bengali, for example: *'Are you in pain?' 'Can I help you?'* and *'Would you like to go to the toilet?'* next to which the English translation can be added, so they can be used during the patient's stay without having to resort to relying on interpreters. This maintains confidentiality, develops the practitioner–client relationship and helps you to meet your duty of care (Ledger 2002), Nursing and Midwifery Council (2008).

- Resources for interpretation and/or translation need to be identified and used when caring for patients who cannot speak English. For example, in order to make information about healthcare more accessible to ethnic minority groups and people who do not speak English, many healthcare trusts provide literature about services and treatment in a number of languages.

- In multicultural and multilingual societies, cue cards or picture boards should be regarded as essential equipment in all areas where patients and clients receive healthcare services. They are used to help clients and patients to describe their symptoms and needs as well as for practitioners to assess care needs, make diagnoses, plan, implement and evaluate care. They are also a means by which practitioners can explain processes and procedures to those in their care.

- There are a number of services available that offer interpretation. Many come under the auspices of the Health Advocacy Services, established by healthcare trusts in the UK. These provide interpreters who are bound by codes of practice. Telephone interpretation services are usually provided by independent agencies. Strict protocols for identifying staff/departments/ organizations using their services are enforced to ensure the confidentiality of patients, clients and others involved. Interpreters for the deaf are available through general interpreting services, primary care trusts as well as through national organizations.

- These services are usually limited and so nurses and midwives need to develop skills such as the effective use of closed questions, perhaps supported by the use of gestures and cue cards or picture boards, which elicit only 'yes' or 'no' answers, so that clients with limited English can express their needs. Staff might have to use their ingenuity by using pens and paper for patients to draw their requirements or for staff to indicate what they are trying to communicate. These circumstances are far from ideal and should never be used if there is a risk of misunderstanding crucial aspects of treatment and care, such as informed consent or clarifying the side-effects of treatment, such as the risk of X-rays in pregnancy.

- In some maternity units, there are specific strategies in place to address this. A 5-year study demonstrated that providing women from minority ethnic communities with a supportive advocate, had a significant effect on maternal and infant health. Volunteer Labour Supporters are women carefully selected and trained in a UK health trust, to support African and Caribbean women during pregnancy and labour. This support has reduced the length of labour and the number of birth interventions. This might be because the women felt more confident when they had the support of an advocate (Tew et al 2006). A number of interventions, aimed at increasing access and engagement with maternity services, for African and African-Caribbean women has been introduced by one large London-based health trust (Walker 2007). The services include bilingual advocacy workers, voluntary supporters in labour and a direct telephone number to talk to a midwife for advice and direction to appropriate services. It is important therefore for professional practitioners to be aware of the services available to promote communication with and support for, those to whom they offer care.

- Remember, those who interpret are legally liable, therefore best practice is always to use a recognized interpreter, rather than an enthusiastic amateur. Family members should be used with caution to protect privacy and confidentiality and ensure accurate interpreting.

Preparation of self

- Consider other situations where you worked with people who do not speak any English. What did you learn from those situations that can inform your practice now?

- If you are male, consider how this might affect Mrs Begum. It might be necessary for you to be chaperoned.

- Consider your feelings. You might be apprehensive about advising Mrs Begum's son that you cannot accept his offer to interpret for his mother. As stated before, acknowledging your feelings and putting them to one side helps to ensure that they do not interfere with the way in which you communicate verbally and non-verbally with mother and son.

- Consider what words you will use to explain the decision not to use her son as an interpreter, so as not to cause him offence. Explain that you will be using the formal interpreting service provided by the hospital.

- Consider how Mrs Begum might be feeling. She is ill and unable to communicate her needs directly. How can you demonstrate empathy and respect to her? You might consider the appropriate use of touch. Perhaps you will offer to shake her hand when you introduce yourself to her.

- Decide the sort of information you need from the son, which will not breach Mrs Begum's confidentiality, such as clarifying the address of her next of kin and the language that she speaks.

- Decide where you will do Mrs Begum's nursing assessment; if you find you might need to use an interpreter, decide which service you require, and check how long it will take before the person can come to the ward. Remember that cultural norms in some ethnic minority communities prefer that women are not interviewed by unknown men unless chaperoned by their husband or a delegated male family member. It is therefore wise to ask for a female interpreter if at all possible.

- Check with other members of the healthcare team whether or not they would also like to use the interpreter when she comes to the ward.

Environment

- Consider the ward environment. Is Mrs Begum's bed in a general ward or in a side room? Is it sufficiently private if you are going to take some time to explain things using an interpreter?

- If you need to employ an interpreter, how much space is there for the nurses and doctors as well as the interpreter to meet around the bed?

- Where are you going to explain to Mrs Begum's son that you cannot use him as his mother's interpreter, without this being overheard or observed? How do you intend to overcome any difficulties of limited space and/or privacy? You might prefer to take Mrs Begum and her son into the ward office or an interview room. Day rooms are usually not private because of their location and design.

Putting the skills into practice

- Approach Mrs Begum with a smile. Introduce yourself by name and offer your right hand to shake hers. Encourage partnership by being friendly and smiling. If her son is there to interpret this encounter, that would be helpful to you all, as it promotes cooperation and mutual respect.

- Wherever this interview is taking place, ensure that her privacy is maintained by closing the door or curtains.

- Assess Mrs Begum's ability to speak English. This could be done by introducing yourself and asking how she is feeling. Use short simple questions.

- Explain to them both that you are working with Mrs Begum today and you are concerned that she understands fully the procedures ahead of her and the care she is to receive. You might like to say: *'I will be working with you today. I want to help you feel comfortable with us and understand about your care.'*

- Explain to her son that you appreciate his thoughtfulness at offering to interpret, but that you will need to use the hospital service. This is because it is important that he is not put in a position where he might have difficulties explaining personal or medical issues.

- Ascertain what language Mrs Begum speaks and explain that you will be getting a hospital interpreter to work with the healthcare team to explain her care to her.

- After ensuring Mrs Begum and her son are clear about what you will be doing, contact the interpreting services, explain the situation and be clear about what language you need to have interpreted and that it would be appropriate to have a woman interpreter. Agree a time when the interpreter will be able to come to the ward and notify the nursing and medical team.

- Inform Mrs Begum and her son about what has been arranged. Relying on the son to interpret could be difficult but if managed sensitively and with respect, it promotes partnership in care.

- When the interpreter arrives introduce her to Mrs Begum and her son. It is preferable to do this before you introduce her to other members of the care team, as she is there primarily for Mrs Begum's benefit, not for the benefit of the professional practitioners.

- After the interpreter has been introduced to her son, escort him to a suitable area where he can wait while his mother is interviewed. Reassure him that you will remain as his mother's chaperone.

- Explain exactly what you want to know from Mrs Begum as part of your nursing assessment. Wait quietly where both Mrs Begum and the interpreter can see you.

- While the interviews are taking place, ensure that Mrs Begum is not crowded. When other members of the healthcare team come to interview Mrs Begum, stay with her as her chaperone and advocate.

- When the interviews and assessments have been finished, ask the interpreter to ask Mrs Begum what else she might like to have explained or clarified. Ask her to say to Mrs Begum that you realize this is a difficult time for her and that you hope she will feel able to ask you and your colleagues for the help she needs.

- Invite Mrs Begum's son to return to be with his mother, and take your leave of them both for the moment. Thank the interpreter for her time and help.

Reflection on practice

Think about a situation where you have cared for someone who spoke little or no English so you needed to use an interpreter.

- Consider how you felt when you first became aware that the patient or client could not speak English. You might have felt anxious that you would not be able to demonstrate adequately warmth, respect, empathy and genuineness to them. You might have felt stressed because the ward was busy and you realized that this situation would take longer than usual to deal with effectively. You might also have been pleased to have the opportunity to deal with a situation like this, as developing the skills to communicate effectively with people who do not speak English is crucial to compassionate professional practice. How did these feelings influence your approach to the person and any relatives present?

- If you had dealt with a similar situation in the past, how did that influence the ways in which you went about making a therapeutic relationship with the patient or client and developing a collaborative relationship with any relatives?

- How successful were you at putting any anxieties you might have had to one side so you could relate respectfully and empathetically to them all? What helped and/or hindered this process?

- How did your thoughts and feelings influence the way you spoke, the language and non-verbal gestures that you chose?

- What thoughts and feelings did you have if you had to explain to any well-meaning friends or relatives the reasons why you would not be using them as interpreters? What language did you use? How did this affect your developing professional relationship with them?

- How did touch influence the way you and the person in your care interacted? Consider their verbal and non-verbal responses to your verbal and non-verbal cues.

- If you organized an interpreting service, how successful were you in ensuring it met the needs of your patient or client and your colleagues? What helped and/or hindered this process?

- When you worked with the interpreter alongside your colleagues, how successful were you in being the patient's or client's advocate, ensuring their privacy, dignity and sense of safety? How did you try to ensure they did not feel crowded or overwhelmed by the number of people involved? What indications were there for you to draw these conclusions?

- What, if anything, would you like to have done differently? What thoughts and feelings have you had about this situation, that have prompted you to consider developing further your communication skills when working with interpreters? How do you intend to build on this experience?

References

Bayles, K., Tomoeda, C., 2007. Cognitive-communication Disorders of Dementia. Plural, San Diego.

Boazman, S., 2003. A time of transition. In: Parr, S., Duchan, J., Pound, C. (Eds.), Aphasia Inside Out: Reflections on Communication Disability. Open University Press, Maidenhead.

Brearley, G., Birchley, P., 1994. Counselling in Disability and Illness, 2nd edn. Mosby, London.

Casson-Webb, A., Wood, M., 2009. Working with a Deaf Intermediary. NewsLI 68, 11–12 (April).

Chapey, R., Hallowell, B., 2001. Introduction to language intervention strategies in adult aphasia. In: Chapey, R. (Ed.), Language Intervention Strategies in Aphasia and Related Neurogenic Communication Disorders, 4th edn. Lippincott Williams and Wilkins, Philadelphia.

Clarke, M., Clarke, J., 2003. Directions without words. In: Parr, S., Duchan, J., Pound, C. (Eds.), Aphasia Inside Out: Reflections on Communication Disability. Open University Press, Maidenhead.

Craddock, E., 1991. Life at secondary school. In: Taypos, G., Bishop, J. (Eds.), Being Deaf: The Experience of Deafness. Continuum, London.

Department of Health, 2009a. Just Checking. Online. Available at: www.justchecking.co.uk/?gclid=CNzp1qKR55kCFQaA3godCDZJQw (accessed 10 April 2009).

Department of Health, 2009b. Living Well With Dementia: A National Strategy. Department of Health, London. Online. Available at: www.dh.gov.uk/en/Publicationsandstatistics/Publications/PublicationsPolicyAndGuidance/DH_094058 (accessed 6 April 2009).

Disability Discrimination Act, 2005. Office of Public Sector Information, OPSI, London. Online. Available at: www.opsi.gov.uk/Acts/acts2005/ukpga_20050013_en_1 (accessed 21 October 2009).

Disability Rights Commission, 2005. The Duty to Promote Disability Equality Statutory Code of Practice England and Wales. The Stationery Office, London. Online. Available at: www.equalityhumanrights.com/Documents/Disability/Public_sector/Disability_equality_duty/Codes_of_practice/DED_code_EnglandWales.pdf (accessed 20 April 2009).

Farrell, G., 1996. Telephoning a nursing department: callers' experiences. Nurs. Stand. 10 (33), 34–36.

Grasha, A.F., 1995. Practical Applications of Psychology, 4th edn. Harper Collins, New York.

Harris, J., 2005. Speech and language therapy. In: Marshall, M. (Ed.), Perspectives on Rehabilitation and Dementia. Jessica Kingsley, London.

Hoff, L.A., Halisey, B., Hoff, M., 2009. People in Crisis: Clinical and Diversity Perspectives, 6th edn. Routledge, London.

Jolley, D., 2005. Why do people with dementia become disabled? In: Marshall, M. (Ed.), Perspectives on Rehabilitation and Dementia. Jessica Kingsley, London.

Ledger, S.D., 2002. Reflections on communicating with non-English-speaking patients. Br. J Nurs. 11 (11), 773–780.

Le May, A., 1998. Empowering older people through communication. In: Kendall, S. (Ed.), Health and Empowerment: Research and Practice. Arnold, London, pp. 91–111.

Lubinski, R., 2001. Environmental systems approach to adult aphasia. In: Chapey, R. (Ed.), Language Intervention Strategies in Aphasia and Related Neurogenic Communication Disorders. 4th edn. Lippincott Williams and Wilkins, Philadelphia.

Norman, I.J., Redfern, S.J., 1997. Mental Healthcare for Elderly People. Churchill Livingstone, Edinburgh.

Nursing and Midwifery Council, 2008. Code of Professional Conduct. Nursing and Midwifery Council, London. Online. Available at: www.nmc-uk.org/aArticle. aspx?ArticleID=3056 (accessed 13 March 2009).

Parr, S., Duchan, J., Pound, C., 2003a. Setting the scene. In: Parr, S., Duchan, J., Pound, C. (Eds.), Aphasia Inside Out: Reflections on Communication Disability. Open University Press, Maidenhead.

Parr, S., Paterson, K., Pound, C., 2003b. Time please! Temporal barriers to aphasia. In: Parr, S., Duchan, J., Pound, C. (Eds.), Aphasia Inside Out: Reflections on Communication Disability. Open University Press, Maidenhead.

Price, D.L., Gwin, J.F., 2007. Pediatric Nursing. Saunders Elsevier, New York.

Quill, T.E., 1995. Barriers to effective communication. In: Lipkin Jr., M., Putnam, S.M., The Medical Interview: Clinical Care, Education, and Research. Springer, New York, pp. 110–121.

Raven, B.H., 1992. A power/interaction model of interpersonal influence: French and Raven thirty years later. J. Soc. Behav. Pers. 7, 217–244.

Richards, L., 2003. Findings from the Multi-agency Domestic Violence Murder Reviews in London. Metropolitan Police Service, London.

Rogers, C., 1957. The necessary and sufficient conditions of therapeutic personality change. J. Consult. Psychol. 21, 95–103.

Ryan, E.B., Giles, H., Bartolucci, R.Y., Henwood, K., 1986. Psycholinguistic and social psychological components of communication by and with the elderly. Lang. Commun. 6, 1–24.

Scrutton, S., 1999. Counselling Older People. Arnold, London.

Tew, J., Gould, N., Abankwa, D., Barnes, H., Beresford, P., Carr, S., Copperman, J., Ramon, S., Rose, D., Sweeney, A., Woodward, L., 2006. Values and methodologies for social research in mental health. National Institute for Mental Health in England and Social Perspectives Network in collaboration with the Social Care Institute for Excellence. Policy Press, Bristol.

Walker, J., 2007. Reducing Infant Mortality Project. Homerton University Hospital. NHS Foundation Trust, London. Online. Available at: www.teamhackney.org/rim_interim_report_october_2007_final_version_with_pictures.pdf (accessed 21 October 2009).

Whaley, L.F., Wong, D.L., 1991. Nursing Care of Infants and Young Children. Mosby, St Louis.

Williams, N.K., Herman, R., Gajewski, B., Wilson, K.B.S., 2009. Elderspeak communication: impact on dementia care. Am. J. Alzheimers Dis. Other Demen. 24 (1), 11–20.

Further reading

Flynn, C., 2009. Working as an intermediary with BSL/English interpreters. NewsLI 68, 12, (April).

Nursing and Midwifery Council, 2009. Guidance for the care of older people. Nursing and Midwifery Council, London.

Stephenson, C., Grieves, M., Stein-Parbury, J., 2004. Patient and Person: Empowering Interpersonal Relationships in Nursing. Elsevier Churchill Livingstone, Edinburgh.

Useful online resources

Age Concern for England, Scotland and Wales. www.ageconcern.org.uk (accessed 20 April 2009).

Alzheimers Society. http://alzheimers.org.uk/site/scripts/home_info.php?homepageID=53 (accessed 20 April 2009).

British Society of Mental Health and Deafness. www.bsmhd.org.uk (accessed 20 April 2009).

Children of Deaf Parents. www.codpuk.org.uk (accessed 20 April 2009).

Equality and Human Rights Commission. www.equalityhumanrights.com/en/Pages/default.aspx (accessed 20 April 2009).

Royal National Institute for Blind People. www.rnib.org.uk/xpedio/groups/public/documents/code/InternetHome.hcsp (accessed 20 April 2009).

Sign Health. www.signhealth.org.uk (accessed 20 April 2009).

UK Council on Deafness. www.deafcouncil.org.uk (accessed 20 April 2009).

8

Managing difficult situations

What should you do?

Am I going
to die?

Do I smell?

Why me?

What shall
I do?

INTRODUCTION

Our experiences as lecturers have revealed that the questions and situations that qualified staff and students find difficult to address, are often those that highlight their lack of skills or those that stimulate incongruence (see Appendix 1). For example, having to withhold information from a patient when you would prefer to disclose it, or being in a caring role but feeling that you cannot help, might lead to inner conflict. Kirschenbaum & Henderson (1990) suggest that anxiety and vulnerability accompany incongruence, and this in turn can be interpreted as the response to being in a difficult situation; this response might be physical and/or psychological. Students classified as difficult, those situations where they felt they did not have the answer to a particular problem or where they found themselves in a situation which took them by surprise.

PRINCIPLES

The making, maintaining and ending of relationships in healthcare can involve the management of situations that challenge our value systems, identify the need for the expansion of our communication skills or have an impact on our personal life.

Self-disclosure

The experience of embarrassment can take many forms; this can include working with people who are significantly similar to or different from us. Being sensitive to the feelings of others is vital, and what is considered sensitive will vary between people and between cultures. By being aware of your own embarrassment or anxiety you are being genuine and, when expressed in moderation, two purposes can be served. First, you are acknowledging what might interfere with the effectiveness of your communication, and by releasing this internal anxiety you can be free to listen to what the person has to say. Second, it might be appropriate to disclose your feelings of anxiety, embarrassment or sadness to the patient, as this will demonstrate to the patient that you are a human being as well as a healthcare practitioner. This demonstration of empathetic understanding might lead, e.g. to the patient's own embarrassment being reduced. It is important however to be sure that the *focus* of the practitioner's self-disclosure is the wellbeing of the person they are caring for, rather than for the release of the intense emotions and thus for the emotional comfort of the practitioner.

In the dynamic of the practitioner–patient/client relationship, the patient or client might need (at an unconscious level) to consider the practitioner to be psychologically stronger than they are. This would enable them to feel confident that the practitioner will be able to meet their needs during their illness/situation. For example a woman in labour might feel increasingly vulnerable and will need the midwife to be 'strong' for her as her labour progresses. While self-disclosure can facilitate the therapeutic relationship, there are times when this intervention might not be in the patient's/client's best interest. For example, if the practitioner responds to the frequent requests for personal information or opinions from the person in their care, the focus of the conversation moves away from the person to the practitioner. This might be an unconscious strategy used by the person to provide some respite from thinking about their own situation; then they might need to be facilitated and supported in thinking about themselves.

Unconditional positive regard

Throughout your communication (both verbal and non-verbal), you will need to enable the patient to feel that whatever they say about their feelings, thoughts and behaviours is acceptable. This demonstration of unconditional positive regard might be difficult, e.g. where the person has a belief that you do not share, or behaves in a way that you feel is unacceptable. This does not mean however that antisocial behaviour, such as sexual harassment or abusive language, is acceptable.

Discussing intimate information and assisting with intimate procedures

You are working in women's health and this placement includes spending time in the women's outpatient clinic. During this time you have been involved in a variety of activities including admitting patients, assisting with intimate examinations and providing postoperative information prior to discharge.

Some issues raised by this scenario:

- The factors that might affect communication when the patient's/client's health status has an impact on their sexual practice and/or their sexuality
- The practitioner and/or the person in their care might be apprehensive about the nature of the chaperone's role
- The patient, client and/or the practitioner might be apprehensive about the examination of genitalia.

Specific principles

- It is essential to be specific when giving and receiving information, especially when discussing sex, sexuality, intimate examinations and procedures. This will reduce the risk of assumptions being made and important areas left unexplored. Omissions or misinformation are more likely to occur if you and/or the patient are experiencing a high level of anxiety or embarrassment.
- Patients may not want to give extensive information about the effect that their illness has on their sexual activity. However, they do need to be reassured about their sexual activity and feel that they are able to discuss such issues, should they wish to do so (Stead et al 2001). Written information is often useful.

- Humour, laughter and touch are useful strategies; however you will need to assess the appropriateness of their use. For some patients, any difficulties they have discussing personal information could relate to feeling judged and not accepted.

Preparation of self

- What type of information is going to be needed? What words will you use to obtain this information?
- How do you feel about asking questions or giving information of such a personal nature?
- How will you record this information? Make sure you have the appropriate documentation, demonstration equipment, e.g. models of anatomy, and information leaflets for completing this.
- Is the patient alone or accompanied by their partner or another person? If the patient is accompanied, the boundaries of confidentiality need to be established.
- How will your feelings affect your body language, tone of voice and your memory?
- From what you know of the patient, how do you think they respond to this type of experience or conversation?

Environment

- Is there a private room available? If not, how are you going to create privacy in the space available to you?
- What facilities are there in the area you are planning to use, e.g. is there a table and resources to draw or write?
- Are there leaflets or other sources of information available?

Putting it into practice

- It is important to develop a therapeutic relationship with the patient as quickly as possible. Behaviours that will facilitate this include establishing eye contact, appropriate smiling and a reassuring, confident approach.
- If the discussion is to take place at the patient's bedside, consider moving to the quieter side of the patient's bed, drawing the curtains and lowering your voice. Clinical tasks such as helping with catheter care might provide good opportunities to discuss related issues.
- One way to demonstrate empathy might be to share how you feel about being asked these questions or having to be examined.
- When interviewing a patient, consider the structure and sequence of your questions and aim to provide an even balance between open and closed questions. It might also be appropriate to use humour; however, care and

sensitivity must be taken into account. The Royal College of Nursing (2001) has produced useful guidelines for considering and incorporating the sexual health needs of patients into everyday professional practice (see Ch. 5).

- In order to demonstrate unconditional positive regard (acceptance), it is important to consider your body language, facial expression and the words you use, should you hear something that you think is unacceptable and in conflict with your own values. This does not mean that you have to agree with what the patient says or does; it might mean that you will have to focus on the patient's needs and rights rather than your personal values.

- You need to explore any unsafe practices the patient mentions and address any missing or inaccurate information.

- While the patient might not need your assistance preparing for a physical examination, it is important that you speak to them and ensure that they are appropriately covered during the procedure. If chaperoning a patient who is lying on a couch, position yourself near the head of the couch. This will enable eye contact to be established and the degree of anxiety, discomfort or pain the patient might be experiencing to be assessed. You can act as an advocate for them by passing this information on to the person examining the patient, to make sure that they are aware and take this into account.

- If the patient engages in any high-risk behaviours, these will need to be explored. For example, if discussing menstruation with a woman who is about to have a hysterectomy, she might say that she hates sanitary towels. However, following a hysterectomy, tampons are not recommended in the immediate postoperative period; sanitary towels reduce the risk of infection and facilitate the accurate assessment of blood loss.

- If the patient is undergoing a procedure that you wish to observe, you should gain consent from them beforehand. The patient might however prefer you to act as their chaperone, rather than use their examination as a learning experience for you (Royal College of Nursing 2002; see also the Royal College of Nursing 2006 guide for vaginal and pelvic examination).

Reflection on practice

Think back to situations where you have assisted patients or women during intimate procedures or assessment.

- How did you help patients or women in your care to feel at ease?
- How did you ensure that you felt at ease?
- What values do you hold that might have a negative effect on your communication?
- Are there any areas that you find it difficult to be more specific about?
- How would you summarize the quality of your interventions? If there are areas that you are dissatisfied with, what steps will you need to take to address them?

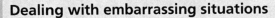

Dealing with embarrassing situations

A student who was recently allocated to the ward was asked to assist a patient out of bed to go to the bathroom. After introducing himself and contracting with the patient (agreeing who would do what), he proceeded to look under the patient's bed for the patient's slippers. After a thorough search he told the patient that he could only find one slipper, to which the patient replied, 'That's because I only have one leg'. The student was so embarrassed that he, 'wished the ground would swallow me up'. The student apologized and the patient laughed, saying that this had often happened. The student then also laughed.

Some issues raised by this scenario:

- The responsibility of the senior practitioner to provide adequate information when delegating a task
- The importance of consulting appropriate documentation before providing care for a patient
- How a mistake might affect the practitioner–patient relationship
- How to re-establish an effective relationship with a patient following a mistake
- How to be open and honest in a therapeutic relationship.

Specific principles

- When a practitioner makes a mistake when caring for a patient or where trust has been breached, the therapeutic relationship will be compromised. Guistolise (1996) and Safran & Muran (1996) identify such incidents as ruptures in the relationship, but reassure us that these can be repaired and might lead to a richer quality of interaction between the patient and the practitioner.
- While humour and laughter are essential components of everyday life, the practitioner needs to make a distinction between 'laughing with' and 'laughing at' the patient and whether or not it is appropriate to laugh at all.

Environment

- The patient was an amputee on a ward and had become increasingly dependent on the nurse to assist with his mobility. In such situations, personal possessions need to be conveniently placed to enable the patient to obtain them as independently as possible. However, the patient might wish an artificial limb to be kept somewhere discreet rather than on view to all.

Putting the skills into practice

- It is important to establish eye contact with the patient and not to laugh alongside the patient following such an incident. It is quite likely that the patient's laugh is what is called a 'gallows laugh' or, in Freudian theory, an unconscious defence known as reaction-formation (see Appendices 1 and 2).

- It is inappropriate to join in with the patient's response to what amounts to a lack of appropriate care; instead, an intervention that includes an apology and demonstrates empathic understanding is required.

- One way to identify an intervention that you feel comfortable using is to consider how you would feel if you were the patient and this type of incident had happened to you on a number of occasions. What would you think about the staff? What response would lead you to feel that the nurse had an understanding of how you were feeling at that moment? For example: *'I am very sorry about that. I imagine you are really annoyed that this keeps happening.'*

- Expressing one's embarrassment at the time of an incident can lead to the relief of any anxiety that is being experienced, and lessen the likelihood of inappropriate expression, in this case 'nervous laughter'. An example of skilled self-disclosure in this situation would have been to apologize and to say something like, *'I'm really embarrassed about making this mistake.'*

- The recognition of the gallows laugh and a verbal reflection of how frustrating it must be (or check with the patient how they feel about this happening), might lead to a more in-depth discussion with the patient about how they feel about being in hospital and their current quality of life. This information can then be shared with appropriate people and the documentation updated as necessary.

Reflection on practice

- In situations where a mistake has been made, it is essential to consider how and why the situation occurred and strategies to prevent something similar happening in the future.

- Does the person in your care appear satisfied with the care they have received and the resolution of any misunderstandings? If not, how are you going to address this?

- Is the patient/client demonstrating signs of anger, frustration or dissatisfaction? If so, what are you going to do? How are you going to defuse the situation?

- What skills do you need to use and how effective are you at putting them into practice?

- In situations similar to the one highlighted in the scenario, who needs to be informed about the interaction? What documentation also needs to be completed?

The psychological importance of similarities and differences in healthcare

While on a ward placement, a Zimbabwean student is asked to assist an elder Zimbabwean male with his hygiene needs.

In this scenario, the similarity of culture is used as a means of considering the impact that similarity (and hence difference) might have on boundaries in the practitioner–patient relationship. It would also be beneficial to consider other similarities such as age, gender, class and status and the impact these might have on the practitioner–patient relationship. The similarity might also be around the use of language and where both share the same first language which is not the dominant language of the country.

The issues addressed include:

- The importance of self-awareness when working with people
- The impact of conscious and unconscious processes on healthcare practice
- Strategies for enhancing the cultural sensitivity of the care provided.

Specific principles

- While working with patients or clients, it is inevitable that preference for some and dislike of others might be experienced. It is important that you develop an awareness of these thoughts and feelings, since they will have an impact on your approach to the people in your care.

- It might be obvious to you why you like or dislike a patient/client, e.g. you might like the fact that they are always polite or have a good sense of humour. However, it might be difficult to pinpoint exactly what it is about them that you find difficult to work with. In such circumstances self-disclosure in a discussion with your mentor, a registered practitioner or your personal tutor might help your unconscious become conscious (see Ch. 1).

- It could be that the patient or situation reminds you of a similar person or past experience and that you are responding in the same way you did to that experience and not to the reality of the current situation. This would be termed transference. In a similar vein, when a patient/client responds to a practitioner in the same way they have done to a previous practitioner who looks similar, e.g. this would be called countertransference (see Ch. 1).

- By identifying that a similarity or difference is having an adverse effect on the practitioner–patient relationship, there is the opportunity to make appropriate adaptations or challenge any assumptions. The following provides an example of how this phenomenon might present and a suggestion for addressing such a situation:

  A patient, who has had a previous admission on another ward, is admitted to your ward. You notice that they appear to be in pain but they have not asked for help. When you mention it the patient says, *'I don't like to bother you. The staff in the last ward were always busy and it seemed as if I was bothering them when I asked for painkillers.'* You reply, *'I'm sorry you felt like that. It's no bother. Please feel free to ask any of us if you need anything. Would you like something for pain now?'* This clarification of the situation provides firmer ground upon which the practitioner–patient relationship can develop.

- While the patient is in your care, there is a need to create a balance between establishing and maintaining a professional relationship and becoming appropriately attached to the patient to enable them to feel 'cared for'.

- In order to reduce the possibility of the patient feeling that you are the only one (because of your similarity) that can provide specific aspects of their care, sharing information with your colleagues is important. If this is not done, an unhealthy dependence can result with the person in your care not expressing their needs until 'their' nurse/midwife arrives. This could also lead to the patient's needs being unmet and appropriate care not being offered.

- It is also important that you challenge and explore any assumptions the patient expresses, e.g. when the patient says, 'You know what I mean'. The patient's assumptions might be based on face value (literally), and your perception based on what you think a person from the same background would want. This might not however reflect the actual needs of the patient and these might remain unmet. The result would be that the patient would be left feeling disappointed, and you left unsure about where you went wrong.

The information that follows is designed to encourage you to think not only of the practical aspects of your work with patients/clients, but also of the psychological factors that will influence the care you provide. This exploration will also help illuminate the personal–professional boundary.

Preparation of self

- What is the nature of your relationship with the patient or client?
- Who do they remind you of?
- Who do you remind them of?
- What assumptions are you aware of making when you encounter people who are similar to, or different from you?
- What type of differences and similarities do you find it more difficult to work with, e.g. older or younger people or people of your own age group? How, if at all, does social class affect your practice?
- What resources (e.g. literature on transcultural healthcare) are available to help you explore the issues you might have raised above?
- What type of differences and similarities do you find it easier to work with?

Environment

- To what extent does the ward environment reflect that to which the person in your care is accustomed in their own country? It would be appropriate to explain the location of various facilities such as the bathroom, and to highlight any of the ward policies. This would be designed to help them become familiar with the environment in order to reduce their anxiety.

- What expectations might the patient/client hold with regard to your role as a professional practitioner and their role as a patient? For example, the patient might not be familiar with the expectation that they can question actions and seek advice from the doctors and other members of the healthcare team; the practitioner might need to clarify these options.

Putting it into practice

- Any similarities that you share with a patient or client might mean that areas such as hygiene practices and religious/spiritual rituals are known and facilitated as much as possible.
- While assisting them with their care, it would be useful to explore their previous experiences of being in hospital in this and other countries.
- It is important that you share this information with colleagues verbally and through documentation.
- While carrying out care and in general conversation with the person in your care, it would be opportune to explore their assumptions based on your appearance, similarities and differences, as a means of gathering information regarding the extent the patient/client feels that their needs are being met.

Reflection on practice

- Think back to a patient or client that you were very fond of. What, if anything, did you find special about this person?
- How do you feel when you provide care for someone who is similar to or different from you (e.g. race, culture, age)?
- Do you treat this person in the same way you treat other patients/clients? If not, why do you think this is?
- What strategies do you think you might need to employ in order to maintain a professional relationship with the person?
- What do you imagine it will be like for you and the patient or client when they, or you, leave the placement?

Dealing with sensitive situations

One of your patients has developed a wound infection and is coming to terms with their altered body image. The patient asks you: 'Do I smell?'

This scenario explores how the health care professional can use the core conditions and effective communication skills while helping a patient to come to terms with altered body image. It invites you to think about how you would address a situation where it is important not to cause offence, and where it is also your responsibility to assist the patient in managing changes in their health.

Specific principles

- Providing information and supporting patients with the consequences of their illness are central parts of your role. At times this might involve giving information that might cause embarrassment, disappointment or concern for you, the patient or both.

- Open and honest communication is a cornerstone of the development and maintenance of an effective therapeutic relationship.

- As a practitioner you can help the patient to develop strategies that can enhance their quality of life, by being willing to take notice of the concerns that they might express. However, some patients might express themselves less directly than others, and more time and skills might be needed to interpret what they are saying.

Preparation of self

- Consider your facial expression and general body language.

- Pay attention to your senses, particularly those of sight and smell. What are they telling you? Is there an odour? How noticeable is it?

- What do you know about how this patient is coping with their health condition?

- What do you imagine their psychological needs might be?

- With this in mind, what is the objective of your communication: to explore the patient's emotional state, to solve the problem of an odour or both?

- How much time do you and the patient have?

Environment

- Where is this interaction taking place? In the bathroom or toilet, at the bedside or while walking along a corridor? The location of this interaction will determine the depth to which you should explore the patient's concern at this point.

- The more privacy that you can offer the patient the more appropriate it will be to discuss the matter in greater depth.

Putting it into practice

- It is important that you remain physically close (or draw nearer to the patient), since their verbal expression indicates a fear of rejection.

- Establish eye contact with the patient and it might also be appropriate to use touch as a therapeutic intervention (Sundeen et al 1998). This will depend on your relationship with the patient and your assessment of their emotional state.

- A genuine response, acknowledging whether there is or is not an odour, will assist the patient in accepting their reality: the patient might exaggerate the intensity of any odour they consider exists, e.g. 'I smell disgusting. I'm sure everyone knows it's me'. The extent of your confirmation might need to be modified. Confirming that there is an odour is important, but knowing that it permeates the whole ward will not help the patient.

- Consider your automatic response and monitor your facial expression, particularly if there is an offensive smell. Although the patient will be listening for your verbal response, it is highly probable that they will be paying more attention to your facial expression. It is therefore essential to ensure that there is congruence between your facial expression and your verbal statement, and that both are appropriate.

- It is also important to take into account the impact the information might have on the patient's self-esteem. Use of empathetic understanding about the reality of their situation might facilitate the move to problem-solving, if appropriate. For example, the practitioner might say, *'You sound very concerned about this. You're right, your wound does smell a little, but it's not as bad as you suggest. I'll change your dressing and use a dressing designed to reduce the smell. Is there anything else that you think might help you feel more comfortable about this?'*

- If there is minimal or no odour at all, it would be appropriate to explore this with the patient rather than dismiss it; e.g. invite the patient to describe what the smell is like. It is possible however that 'the smell' might be a façade for other anxieties or concerns that the patient might have, but finds it difficult to discuss. In such circumstances, by raising this issue of a smell, the patient has attracted your attention and it is now your job to facilitate them in revealing their concerns.

- Depending on your relationship with the patient, it might be appropriate to use the skill of advanced empathy, and offer them an interpretation of what you think is going on. For example, *'I can see that you are worried. I wonder if it's about your treatment/having surgery/being discharged.'*

- If a patient complains repeatedly of an odour that is minimal or does not exist, this might be their way of expressing another underlying anxiety. It is important that you treat this defence with respect. In this situation you can either provide regular assurance that there is no odour or choose to explore the underlying anxiety in more depth.

- It is, however, inappropriate to deny the existence of an odour if an odour does exist, particularly if this is done because it is thought that it would be unkind to tell the truth. Interventions such as, 'Of course not' or 'We're used to it', are blocks to further interaction on the subject and therefore inhibit the development of a meaningful therapeutic relationship.

- As a nurse or midwife, being used to a sight, sound or a smell is part of becoming a professional practitioner; however, as a means of conveying the uniqueness of a particular patient, their experience and your recognition of how they may be feeling, it is not a useful intervention. A further consequence of such interventions is that they deny the opportunity for the enhancement of problem-solving and communication skills in both you and the person in your care.

- Depending on their needs, the above interventions might be useful in helping allay the patient's concerns about offending you. It is important to remember, however, that **protecting you** should not be the concern of the patient.

- If the environment is not conducive to in-depth exploration (e.g. while accompanying the patient to another department), acknowledge that there is an issue that needs to be addressed and contract with the patient for a time and place when you will speak with them about the issue. It is important to ensure that you keep to that commitment.

- At the end of your interaction it would be beneficial to summarize the areas of discussion and reflect (both verbally and non-verbally) your appreciation of the patient's level of concern.

Reflection on practice

When faced with unexpected situations, it might be difficult to know what to say for the best, or how to say it. Each time you are faced with such situations, it is useful to reflect upon how you managed them. It is also useful to consider discussing the 'what would I say if' scenarios with your mentor.

- If you were in a similar situation, to what extent do you feel you would be able to demonstrate acceptance of the patient? What evidence do you have to support your answer?

- How might you improve your use of empathetic understanding?

- Have there been times when you have felt stuck during an interaction with a patient? If so, why do you think this happened?

- What skills do you need to develop further?

- What have you learnt that might be applied to other patients and future clinical placements?

Withholding information

One of the patients on your ward is terminally ill and wants to know what is wrong with them and asks you if they are going to die. Although you want to be honest with the patient and give them the information, it was made clear in the handover and in the patient's notes that the patient was not to be told their diagnosis. You are very uncomfortable about this.

Some issues raised by this scenario:
- The importance of reflection
- Strategies to be used to ensure the maintenance of an effective therapeutic relationship in such a situation.

Specific principles

- When working in a team or in an organization, there will be times when decisions are made which go against one's personal philosophy, but with which one has to conform. This scenario explores a situation where the agreed strategy is to withhold information regarding diagnosis from the patient. Although it is important that the nurse is familiar with the legal and ethical issues surrounding such a decision, this is not the focus of the following discussion.

- Interactions with the patient might be strained, particularly if the nurse is experiencing inner conflict (incongruence) caused by a desire to tell the patient and an instruction not to do so.

- The interventions might focus on how to remain within the agreed protocol for the patient, but the strain on open and honest communication might be compounded if the patient is anxious or distressed by the lack of information.

- It is important that the healthcare team is able to negotiate and agree the plan of care. However, each team member might belong to a different hierarchical structure, and values and beliefs might clash (Roberts 1994). Occasionally, where beliefs differ, acceptance of the situation is necessary.

- Reflecting on a given situation from the perspective of each person concerned will provide valuable insights and this might make acceptance easier to manage and work with. Being aware of your feelings about a given situation and being able to put the distracting elements aside is an essential skill for all healthcare practitioners. It is equally important that you have another forum within which these distracting thoughts and feelings can be explored. The ward meeting, a tutorial, clinical supervision or reflection sessions are examples of appropriate arenas for this activity.

- In such a situation, it is difficult if the patient asks about their diagnosis. 'We're all going to die' is sometimes suggested as an appropriate response but, while this is certainly the truth, this response is unlikely to meet the emotional or cognitive needs of the patient. The maintenance of a therapeutic relationship is also threatened since such interventions do not encourage the patient to discuss how they feel about their situation.

- The use of such responses reflects one of two things: either a lack of awareness or the level of anxiety experienced by the nurse in the face of such a question. The response could be considered as a defence against this anxiety, since it blocks the depth of conversation that the patient desires.

- At times other strategies might also be used to reduce anxiety, such as ignoring the question, changing the subject or using humour. While the use of humour in the clinical setting is often useful, the nurse needs to consider the appropriateness of this intervention.

Preparation of self

- Why do you think the patient needs to know their diagnosis? What do you imagine their needs are at this time?
- What thoughts and feelings did you have when the patient asked you these questions?
- What thoughts and feelings do you have about withholding the information?
- What is your assessment of the patient's psychological state? How does this assessment contribute to your interactions with the patient?
- Has the patient asked other members of staff or are you the only one they have asked?
- What do you know about the information that is being withheld? How long will the information be withheld?
- What do you know about this patient's spiritual, religious and cultural beliefs?
- If you were able to speak openly and honestly with the patient, what would you say?
- What areas do you think this discussion will lead to? Have you discussed these areas before? Do you feel you have the necessary skills to support the patient as they explore these issues or do you need the support of a more experienced practitioner?
- If unable to discuss the patient's diagnosis, what other aspects of the patient's care or situation could you explore, rather than avoiding the patient?
- Who have you consulted to express your concerns and to provide support for you in this situation?

Environment

- In such situations, it is useful to note what was happening immediately prior to being confronted with this situation, as this might be an indication of the patient's level of anxiety. For example, were you assisting the patient with an aspect of their care or were you simply passing by their bed?
- Is there anyone else with the patient or are they alone? If they are with a relative, it might be the relative that is forcing the issue.

Putting the skills into practice

- Consider your automatic response and monitor your facial expression, particularly if this request has taken you by surprise. It might be appropriate to disclose that you were surprised by the question.
- It is important that you remain physically close or move nearer to the patient. This will reflect that you understand the seriousness of the question and will also act as a means of providing privacy.

- Establish eye contact with the patient and, depending on your relationship with them and your assessment of their emotional state, it might be appropriate to use touch as a therapeutic intervention.

- The environment within which the issue is raised might not be conducive to in-depth exploration, i.e. you are in the process of doing a wound dressing or you are helping the patient while in the toilet. It is crucial to acknowledge that they have raised important issues that need to be discussed and agree a time and a place where this discussion can take place. It would also be appropriate to mention if you are going to speak with another member of the healthcare team about their concerns.

- The above strategy serves two purposes: first, it protects the patient's privacy and self-esteem by planning for the discussion to take place in a more secure environment; and second, it provides time for both you and the patient to think about the next step.

- The patient might feel some relief about the fact that they have raised the issue and might now need some time to think about what they are going to say. They might also wish to contact a member of their family or a friend to ask them to visit. The nurse can also take this opportunity of time to seek advice, consult another member of the team and think about what future actions might be appropriate.

- Alternatively, the environment might be where such a conversation can take place, where a degree of privacy can be assured, where the patient can be comfortable and where appropriate verbal and non-verbal communication can take place.

- In responding to direct or implied questions like, 'Am I going to die?' you have a number of options. One is to respond with empathic understanding (see Ch. 4), e.g. *'I can see that you look worried'* and this could be followed with open focused encouragement such as, *'Tell me more about how you have been feeling lately.'*

- The skill of active listening involves listening to what is unspoken as well as the spoken word. For a greater understanding of this, imagine the thoughts and feelings you would have if you were being asked either of the above questions.

- For example, the patient might speak at length about the impact of their illness on a family member, but not mention how they are feeling. Addressing this with the patient will depend on your skills, your relationship with the patient and the appropriateness of the location.

- It might be that the patient signals (verbally or non-verbally) that they do not wish to talk about a particular issue. While you might feel discouraged about this, you have signalled to the patient that you have noticed something important and that you are available to discuss it, should they wish to.

- Specific responses reflecting the patient's condition might also be appropriate, e.g. *'It does seem as if your symptoms are taking a long time to respond to the treatment.'* Open questions such as, *'What do you think is wrong with you?'* or *'How do you think you are progressing?'* will imply your willingness and ability to engage with the client at a very personal level, therefore such interventions should not be used unless this is your intention.

- However, since this might be exactly the type of conversation that the patient wants to have with a member of the team, you could say, *'It sounds as if you want to be clear about what is wrong with you'* or *'It sounds as if you are very concerned that you are not getting better.'* Either statement could then continue: *'I'm not able to discuss these issues with you, but I will ask the nurse in charge/doctor to come and speak with you urgently. In the meantime is there anything I can do for you now?'*

- There are occasions when a patient feels out of control, helpless and/or powerless. It is helpful if you are aware of this and use interventions that offer choices, encourage the patient and help boost their self-esteem. For example, *'It certainly sounds as if you have been giving this a lot of thought. Would you like to talk to the doctor about your thinking?'*

- It would be appropriate for you to accompany the team member who will subsequently speak with the patient, since the patient has established a relationship with you. However, it would be respectful to seek permission from the patient first.

- At the end of your interaction it is beneficial to summarize the areas of discussion and reflect (both verbally and non-verbally) your appreciation of the patient's level of concern.

- If a senior member of staff was not present during your discussion, it would be important to update them on what has been said, and inform your colleagues in the next handover. Completion of appropriate documentation will ensure that the team is conversant with the latest developments with regard to the patient's concerns and the information that the patient has.

Reflection on practice

Think back to a situation where you have been unable to disclose information, such as test results to a patient.

- How would you monitor the changes in a patient's psychological state during such an interaction?

- How effective are you in supporting patients through this type of experience?

- How might you improve your use of empathic understanding?

- Have there been occasions during an interaction when you have not known what to say?

- What have you learnt about communicating with patients experiencing such uncertainty? What skills do you need to develop further?

- What have you learnt that could be applied to other patients and future clinical placements?

- What support do you need to be able to reflect on such situations? Are there any changes that you need to make to your support network?

Supporting a pregnant woman in decision-making

A woman has been in hospital for over a week having various tests and scans and is awaiting the results. She asks the midwife, *'Why me?'* or *'What would you do?'*

This scenario reflects some of the fundamental existential questions that practitioners might face, but that cannot be answered, other than by acknowledging the feelings that often accompany them. These questions might also be difficult because the practitioner has not explored them with regard to their own lives and circumstances.

Some issues raised by this scenario:

- How to use self-disclosure effectively
- How to inform and give advice efficiently
- How to manage one's own anxiety and help the person in your care manage their anxiety.

Specific principles

- Maintaining a balance between personal and professional relationships might be difficult at times, particularly if the practitioner identifies closely with the patient or woman's situation and finds it hard to maintain the distinction between themselves and the patient.

- Deciding if, when and how to disclose personal information to a person in your care is a challenging skill, since in some situations it can significantly enhance the relationship. However, in other situations the person might consider it an unwanted intrusion.

- Enabling patients and clients to make their own decisions is often more difficult than telling them what to do for the best, and it might also be more time-consuming. There are clearly times when it is the practitioner's role to let the woman know what might be in their best interest, e.g. *'You will probably find it easier to breathe if you have a few more pillows supporting your back. I'll go and get some for you.'* There are others, however, when you cannot make the decision for the person in your care; such as a pregnant woman, when discussing the option of the administration of Vitamin K to her baby after delivery, might ask you, *'What would you do?'*

- At times, practitioners are very focused on problem-solving and use this as their primary and main intervention, particularly in the face of staff shortages. Moving to problem-solving might also be a strategy for reducing anxiety when faced with the reality of not knowing what to do or say. Silence might be an appropriate option. (For a useful framework which identifies the choices we have when communicating, see Heron 2001).

- Lack of experience or awareness might also cause the practitioner to take the patient's or client's questions literally and begin the search for answers; when 'staying with' and supporting them might be the best solution.

Preparation of self

- Why do you think the woman is asking the question?
- What thoughts and feelings do you have when women or patients ask questions such as these?
- As you listen and observe women or patients, how do you assess their psychological state?
- How does this assessment affect your interactions with the person in your care?
- Are you the only person that the woman or patient has asked, or have other members of staff been approached? It is important that the woman or patient does not develop an unhealthy reliance on you.
- What would you like to say to them? How do you imagine this might help or hinder them?
- What do you know about your client's or patient's spiritual, religious and cultural beliefs?
- In light of the information that you have about your clients/patients regarding their health, what other resources and information would be useful for you to consult?

Environment

- What was happening immediately prior to being confronted with the situation? For example, were you assisting the woman with an aspect of her care or were you simply passing by her bed, or has she just been seen by the doctors?
- Knowledge of what preceded the woman's statement might provide you with a reference point from which to begin your interaction. For example, if this occurred while assisting a woman with her hygiene needs, you might explore the impact her pregnancy is having on her independence and how she feels about this. It might be that other strategies or resources might need to be employed, especially if the woman is due to be discharged.
- Where is this interaction taking place? In the bathroom or toilet? At the bedside? In the corridor? The location of this interaction will determine the depth to which the concern can be addressed.
- It is important that you remain physically close (or draw nearer to the patient), since this will afford the person some privacy and show them that you are paying attention.
- Establish eye contact with the patient and it might also be appropriate to use touch as a therapeutic intervention. This will depend on your relationship with the woman and your assessment of their emotional state.

- A genuine response, acknowledging the dilemma or situation they are facing, would be appropriate.

- If the environment is not conducive to in-depth exploration, acknowledge that you hear their concern and contract with the person in your care for a time and place when you will talk about the issue. It would also be appropriate to mention if you intend to inform another member of the healthcare team about their concerns.

- The above strategy serves two purposes: first, it protects the person's privacy and self-esteem by planning for the discussion to take place in a more secure environment and second, it provides time for both the practitioner and the person to think about the next stage.

- The woman might feel some relief about the fact that she has raised the issue and might now need some time to think about what she is going to say. She might also wish to contact a member of her family or a friend to ask them to visit. The nurse/midwife can take this opportunity of time to seek advice, consult another member of the team and think about what future actions might be appropriate.

- Alternatively, the environment might be one within which such a conversation can take place, that is, where a degree of privacy can be assured, where the woman or patient can be comfortable and where appropriate verbal and non-verbal communication can take place.

- In responding to direct or implied questions like, 'Why me?', the practitioner has a number of options. One is to respond with empathetic understanding, 'I can see that you look worried.' This might be followed with an open question, 'Tell me more about how you have been feeling lately.'

- 'Why me?' might also be a verbal exclamation to the woman's or patient's spiritual/religious being. One way to demonstrate respect if this is the case, would be to witness the expression, remain silent but use your body language to show you recognize the despair that they might be experiencing. For example, sit with them, hold their hand and adjust your facial expression. An appropriate verbal response might be, 'Yes, you are having a rough time.'

- Aiming to answer such a question might leave both participants dissatisfied, therefore it would be best to try and capture the feelings that underpin such statements. At times there are occasions when a woman or patient feels out of control, helpless, hopeless and powerless. It is useful for the practitioner to be aware of this and use interventions and offer choices that encourage the person and help them boost their self-esteem.

- Active listening involves listening to what is unspoken as well as the spoken word. For a greater understanding of this, it would be useful to imagine the thoughts and feelings you would have if you were asking either of the questions asked by the woman.

- It might be beneficial to sit with the woman or patient and listen without offering solutions. Silence will facilitate listening and allow them to feel free to speak. Occasional reflection and paraphrasing might be used as appropriate. For example, *'It is unfair that you are having to suffer like this'* or *'It is really frustrating not knowing what to do for the best. I can't tell you what to do but I am here to support your decision and give you what information I can.'* This would enable the person to tell their story and give the practitioner a clear picture of the woman's or patient's perspectives and concerns.

- An example of a response using self-disclosure and reflecting the woman's dilemma might be, *'When I was faced with a difficult decision recently I found it useful to write down the pros and cons of the options and then I discussed these with …'* or *'I really don't know what I would do if I were in your situation. I'd hope there were people around to help me and I guess I'd make a decision eventually, but I know it wouldn't be easy. This is why we're here, to give you information and support you in making your decision and open focused.'*

- Open questions and open focused questions such as, *'What do you think would be the best for you?'* or *'What choices do you feel you have?'* are interventions that will give the signals to the patient that you are willing and able to engage in helping them. These are examples of what Heron (2001) terms catalytic interventions.

- If the woman has inaccurate or insufficient information, agree a strategy for addressing this. For example, it might be appropriate to teach her (see Ch. 10) to obtain other resources or arrange for a specialist practitioner or other member of the healthcare team to visit.

- At the end of your interaction it is beneficial to summarize the areas of discussion and reflect (both verbally and non-verbally) your appreciation of how concerned the person is.

- If it has been arranged for another member of the team to visit the woman, it would be appropriate for you to accompany them when they speak with her, since the patient has established a relationship with you. However, it would be respectful to seek permission from the woman first.

Reflection on practice

Think of a similar situation in which you have been involved.

- How effective have you been in supporting patients or clients through similar experiences?

- To what extent do you feel you are able to demonstrate acceptance of their perceptions of their situation? What evidence do you have to support your answer?

- How might you improve your use of empathetic understanding?

- Have there been situations where you have not known what to say for the best?

- What have you learnt about the patient/client?

- What have you learnt that might be applied to other patients or clients and future situations?

- What skills do you need to develop further?
- What additional resources did you consult or could you have consulted to facilitate your work with patients and clients facing difficult situations?
- What support did you need at times like these? How effective was the support that you received? Are there any changes that you need to make to your support network?

References

Guistolise, P., 1996. Failures in the therapeutic relationship: inevitable and necessary? Transactional Analysis Journal 26 (4), 284–288.

Heron, J., 2001. Helping the client: a creative practical guide. Sage, London.

Kirschenbaum, H., Henderson, V., 1990. The Carl Rogers Reader. Constable, London.

Roberts, V., 1994. Conflict and collaboration: managing intergroup relations. In: Obholzer, A., Roberts, V. (Eds.), The Unconscious at Work: Individual and Organizational Stress in the Human Services. Routledge, London, pp. 187–196.

Royal College of Nursing, 2006. Vaginal and Pelvic Examination: guidance for nurses and midwives. RCN, London.

Royal College of Nursing, 2002. Chaperoning: The Role of the Nurse and the Rights of Patients. RCN, London.

Royal College of Nursing, 2001. RCN Sexual Health Strategy. RCN, London.

Safran, J., Muran, J., 1996. The resolution of ruptures in the therapeutic alliance. J. Consult. Clin. Psychol. 64 (3), 447–458.

Stead, M., Fallowfield, L., Brown, J., Selby, P., 2001. Communication about sexual problems in ovarian cancer: qualitative study. Br. Med. J. 323, 836–837.

Sundeen, S.J., Stuart, G., Rankin, E.A.D., Cohen, S.A., 1998. Nurse–Client Interaction: Implementing the Nursing Process. Mosby, St Louis.

Further reading

Buckman, R., 2001. Communication skills in palliative care: a practical guide. Neurol. Clin. 19 (4), 989–1004.

Evans, D., 2000. Speaking of sex: the need to dispel myths & overcome fears. Br. J. Nurs. 9, 650–655.

Heath, H., White, I. (Eds.), 2002. The Challenge of Sexuality in Health Care. Blackwell Science, Oxford.

9

Working in groups and teams

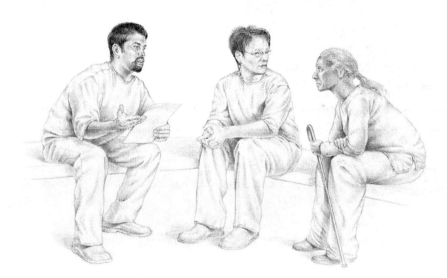

INTRODUCTION

One of the key elements of healthcare practice is the ability to work in a team. 'A team is a small number of people with complementary skills who are committed to a common purpose, performance goals, and approach for which they hold themselves mutually accountable' (Katzenbach and Smith 1993). Larson & LaFasto (1989: 19) define a team as having 'two or more people; it has a specific performance objective or recognizable goal to be attained, and co-ordination of activity among members of the team is required for the attainment of the team goal or objective'. Comparative analysis undertaken by Larson & LaFasto (1989) revealed eight characteristics of effectively functioning teams. These are summarized in Box 9.1.

Referring specifically to healthcare teams, Prosser (2005) considers that effective teams have:

- a clear sense of purpose and direction
- openness as a key characteristic
- a balanced membership
- performance as their main focus of attention
- an effective leader who adopts an appropriate leadership style.

The foundations and principles that can facilitate a team working effectively as shown in Box 9.1 are the same as working within a group, therefore in this chapter

---

Box 9.1 Characteristics of functioning teams (Larson & LaFasto 1989)

Teams that function effectively:
- have clear goals that make a significant difference, i.e. benefit society in some way
- are results-driven, with the resources available to facilitate meeting the goal/objective
- have competent members
- demonstrate a unified commitment
- contain a collaborative climate
- have identified expected standards of excellence
- offer support and recognition to each other
- have a leader who has a clear vision of the result of the goal/objective and who is able to pass this on to the group members. The leader also has the ability to create change; this will also include facilitating others in meeting their potential.

the terms 'team' and 'group' will be used interchangeably. One of the challenges that you face as a student, is the movement from one practice placement to another throughout your course. This frequent movement requires the student to become skilled in initiating, maintaining and ending relationships with members of a team that is already established. In addition, the practice placements might involve different geographical locations, which might add to the unfamiliarity and stress experienced by you, as a result of the time needed to adjust.

The ward culture, staffing levels and frequent change of students allocated to the placement will all contribute to the reception the student receives and might have an effect on their ability to feel and become part of the team. For example, some team members might feel that it is not worth investing time in teaching students who are 'passing through', particularly if the placements are very busy. It is also possible that the frequent change in students allocated to the area is experienced as stressful. The conscious and unconscious perceptions and experiences of both the student and the other members of the team are a major contributing factor in influencing how each gets on with the other. For example, current students might be compared with the previous group of students, without specific experience of how this group behaved.

PRINCIPLES

'The ability to work effectively with a group of other people, either as a leader or member, is an important interpersonal skill' (Hayes 2002: 60). Effective communication increases our ability to provide good-quality care, and enhances our learning potential. Communication in healthcare takes place within the context of an organizational structure that might contain power or hierarchical elements that determine how communication is carried out. Bradley & Edinberg (1982) provide a good discussion of the different communication patterns that exist within healthcare teams.

GROUPS

Where a hierarchy exists, a coalition is essential in order to enhance the quality of communication. When we join a group, there is a need to feel accepted, to feel able to communicate openly and honestly, to express our needs and to receive empathetic understanding about what these needs are. Where these elements form the foundation of the relationship, we are more likely to achieve our potential (Rogers 1961). Through collegiate relationships, members of a group can give each other feedback about how others see us.

Factors contributing to group process and roles

A review of the literature reveals that the evolution of a group is similar to life development: it begins with a high degree of infantile dependence, moves to a stage of rebellion, which involves achieving a sense of identity in the group, and then works to attain greater stability and adult functioning. In other words, groups follow a recognized process of development, which begins with an increased dependence on the person identified as the leader and moves to a position of being able to work autonomously as well as in collaboration with others.

A number of authors (Baron & Kerr 2003, Belbin 2003, Sundeen et al 1998, Clarkson 1993, Yalom 1970, Berne 1966, Tuckman 1965, Bion 1961) have written extensively about these processes, as well as the various roles that individuals adopt when in a group, some of which enhance the effectiveness of the group. It is important to remember when considering stage theories (such as Tuckman's) that a number of factors influence the process, e.g. a group might regress to an earlier stage when a new member joins or someone leaves. A group might also become fixed at a particular stage and might need assistance to move on. For example, if a group is stuck at the storming stage, it is difficult for the task to be addressed, as the atmosphere might not facilitate effective communication. One aspect of an effective healthy group, is that they are able to discuss those aspects that are causing concern as well as the 'nice things'. The roles that contribute to the dynamics of the group can be divided into task and maintenance activities. Task roles include titles such as initiator, consensus taker and summarizer. Maintenance roles include encourager, compromiser and harmonizer.

In a group there will be times when self-protective behaviours are used. For example, one person might be so quiet in the group that they are 'invisible' or in contrast another might be the 'intellectualizer' and tend to overcomplicate the situation and use unnecessarily complex terms. Both of these actions might act as a block to interacting with others in order to control anxiety and maintain self-esteem. Berne (1966) uses the term **IMAGO** (see below) to outline the perceptions we might have before meeting the group and the subsequent process of becoming a group member. Napper & Newton's (2000) contribution to this idea is summarized in Box 9.2.

Box 9.2 **Becoming a group member (adapted from Napper & Newton 2000)**

- **I**magine how the group will be: this will be based on conscious and unconscious past experiences of being in a group and perceptions of the group.
- **M**eet the others and begin to differentiate between them, transferring expectations on to them.
- **A**ngling for one's place in the group might mean accepting a role that is familiar but not necessarily desired.
- **G**et **O**n with each other in the present, without the previous expectations that were projected on to group members. At this point there is open communication in the group and a sense of belonging is experienced.

Group members need to be familiar with the various roles required of an effective group and to become skilled in recognizing the roles that might be missing in a group and modify their behaviour accordingly. For example, group members might be very focused on the task but leave each encounter feeling that their efforts are unappreciated. It might be that no one is occupying the encourager role, which involves (among other things) giving empathetic responses and helping to maintain motivation. It might well be that the placement area has a culture of withholding this type of nurturing from the staff; this might however have a negative effect on the degree of effort that will be put into the group activity. As the group size increases, less effort and investment is put into an activity; Latane et al (1979) call this 'social loafing'.

Working in groups

Increasingly, the nature of healthcare education involves working in groups, in order to explore in greater depth and apply to practice, the theoretical and clinical principles that have been introduced in a lead lecture. This is also taking place with students of other disciplines in healthcare. Introducing project work for groups to undertake has the benefit of enabling you to use the knowledge you already have to explore those gaps in your knowledge. This process can be initiated by the lecturer, e.g. by presenting a patient scenario or an aspect of healthcare, which is then explored by the group with the aim of developing their knowledge and presenting this in a seminar at a later date.

Once the group agrees on what is already known and what information needs to be gathered in order to address the task, the group identifies what further information is needed and allocates various aspects to each group member. The learning process usually culminates with each group presenting the findings of their project to the rest of the cohort in whichever format they feel is appropriate and interesting.

Working in a group

You have just begun another module and during the study week preceding your placement your seminar group has been given a project. At the end of the module, in 12 weeks' time, your group will be expected to present the completed project to the other groups in your cohort. As a group, you need to identify the task and agree the strategies for producing the work before you all leave to go on your placements. There is a session in 4 weeks' time when the group will be expected to present the material they have developed so far.

The scenario above provides the opportunity for you to consider the factors that enable a group to work together in a productive way. It also invites you to think about your behaviour and contributions in groups.

Some issues raised by this scenario:

- Role negotiation and decision-making
- Seeking clarification
- Summarizing
- Challenging.

Specific principles

- Since nursing and midwifery are professions that require practitioners to be able to work in a group or team, one of the benefits of project work is that it provides an opportunity for students to develop the skills of working together. In the early stages of group formation, there is increased dependence on the lecturer/facilitator to make decisions and give instructions.

- As a group progresses, members need to take on the various roles necessary to help the group function in a healthy manner. This will result in less dependence on the lecturer/facilitator for instruction; who can then act as a guide and consultant offering suggestions and/or expert information as appropriate.

- The role of the lecturer therefore moves to become one of a facilitator, not a director. The group might also request that the facilitator provides feedback to them on how they are working together.

- The group (including the facilitator) will need to explore and agree how the group is going to be run and what each expects from the other. This might include such issues as attendance at future meetings or how to address non-participation in the activities by some members of the group.

- If this is the first time the group has met or they have not worked together before in this way, the facilitator is likely to introduce some team-building activities in order to aid this process. This would also be appropriate if there has been a change in the group make-up.

- One of the skills of working in a group is being able to recognize how the behaviour of the group members (including oneself) affects the group's performance and achievement of the identified goals.

- Another feature of an effective group is that, once the agreed goal has been achieved, the group is psychologically able to move on to work efficiently on another project. Debriefing and reflection can facilitate this.

- Equally important is the ability to appreciate the knowledge and skills each person in the group has, and when engaged in group activity, encourage the appropriate use of the skills in a non-manipulative way (see also Ch. 6).

- Care needs to be taken with regard to decision-making and allocation of tasks in a group. This is because the status or verbosity of an individual might be the criteria that are used for selection, rather than the appropriate matching of their expertise for the task. Task allocation might be an opportunity for another member of the group to develop their skills.

- A group is likely to work best if they consider the task to be relevant to their personal goals and whether or not the task provides an appropriate level of difficulty.

- As the group size increases, the investment in the task might diminish, therefore subgroups need to be practical and enable appropriate communication.

- Where a group is very concerned about maintaining a smooth easy-going atmosphere, particularly in the 'storming' stage of development (Tuckman 1965), this can inhibit creativity and result in the group agreeing on the one or two ideas that have been generated. Larson & LaFasto (1989) call this 'groupthink'. Exploring this process and introducing other possibilities will help the group members move towards a more rewarding and productive experience. It might be useful to refer to Chapter 6 and Figures A1–4 for additional information.

Preparation of self

- What is your understanding about what is expected of the project/topic?
- How do you feel about being in this seminar group?
- How does this affect your work and communication in the group?
- What are your personal goals and how do they fit in with the goals of the group?
- What role(s) do you think you might take during this group activity? Is this how you want to participate in this group?
- Are there any particular parts of the project that you would like to work on?
- Which of the group members would you particularly like to work with? What are your reasons for this?
- Which of the group members do you think it might be difficult to work with? Why do you think this would be the case? What might you gain by working with them?

Environment

- Is the environment conducive to the discussion that you need to have in order to ensure you all understand what is expected? Will group members be able to meet while on your various placements? What other suitable locations might there be?

- Are there appropriate resources available for you to engage in identifying the relevant issues and planning the way forward? For example, would it be useful for you to have a flip chart or whiteboard, pens, contact details, books, articles or a diary to record dates for future meetings?

Putting the skills into practice

- Listen to the information that is being given regarding the project and seek clarification about exactly what your group is expected to do.

- Ensure that you contribute to the discussion about how the group is going to function, particularly if something is suggested and you are unsure or unhappy about what is expected or assumed about your participation.

- If you decide that you would like to contribute more or less than you usually do in the group, it would be useful to outline this to the other members, so that they can adjust their expectations of you.

- Once you have decided upon your personal objectives for this module, consider how the project might contribute to this. It would be useful to express your preference and find out who else has similar interests.

- Aim to be realistic in the amount of work you agree to do. This will involve setting limits to ensure that there is equity in the group. Being clear about what you are willing to do will also lessen the likelihood of sabotaging the success of the group by consciously or unconsciously 'forgetting' to do something (see Ch. 6).

- Ensure that you summarize any tasks that you have agreed to do.

Reflection on practice

Think back to your experiences of working as part of a group or team.

- When engaging in group work, what is your level of concentration and participation in the group like? What affects your ability to listen and participate?

- How would you sum up your relationship with the other members of the group?

- What type of contributions do you make in this group? For example, are you the one who makes suggestions? Is your primary aim to seek agreement among the group or are you the 'invisible' person?

- Do you feel able to ask someone else, who appears to have the appropriate knowledge and skills, to undertake a task that is being suggested?

- When you have been part of a group but you have not contributed to the decisions that have been made, how do you feel about that?

- When in a group and seeking clarification, do you feel you have a clear understanding about the work that is to be carried out? If not, how can this information be obtained more effectively?

- When you think back to the first time you were in your seminar group, how did you feel? What did you think of it? How has your opinion altered?

- As you reflect on the variety of groups that you have belonged to or still belong to (e.g. ward team, student group, church/social groups), how does your participation in each vary? In what way might you need to increase or decrease your involvement in order to achieve your goals in a healthy manner?

When others do not pull their weight

You are back in your university for a study day and your seminar group is scheduled to have a session in order to give feedback to each other regarding the activities that have been agreed in the first study week. As the session progresses it becomes clear that, while you have made an effort to do some of the work you agreed to do, some of the others have not.

Some issues raised by this scenario:

- Assessing the team atmosphere
- Recognizing and addressing conflict
- Giving and receiving feedback
- Paraphrasing
- Using humour.

Specific principles

- If an individual does not identify with the group (they might feel excluded or have excluded themselves) they are likely to put little effort into the group task. To increase effectiveness this needs to be addressed.

- If there is a strong group identity, members are more likely to have a greater commitment to the success of the group. This would contribute to the motivating force of healthy competition with any other seminar groups.

- Some people, for a variety of reasons, find it difficult to contribute in a group. However, the consequence is that they deprive others in the group from being able to learn from them, and might not make themselves available to learn from others.

- There is always a need in a group for each member to pay attention to their own and others' experiences of being in the group. This will include aspects such as how empathetic members are, how feedback is given and received and how the accomplishments of group members are acknowledged.

  Note: It might be useful to refer to Chapter 6 for more details.

Preparation of self

- In situations where you have realized that some of your colleagues had not done the work they had agreed to, how do you feel?

- In light of this, what feedback do you want to give the group or the individual about this?

- Having considered how you have felt or might feel and what you think, how are you going to give this information in a way that maintains respect for yourself and for the other person?
- Having considered the work that you have done, how are you going to present your contribution in a concise manner?

Putting the skills into practice

- In discussing your group, it is useful to use inclusive words such as 'us', 'we' and 'our'. This not only provides a sense of belonging and cohesiveness but might be experienced as non-blaming by the person with whom you are speaking.
- A greater sense of achievement can be attained if you develop the skill of offering help and asking for it when you need it.
- It might be appropriate to speak to the person individually or generalize the feedback if it is an issue that is a common feature of the group. For example, although one person might be persistently late, lateness might be a major feature of the group.
- State the issue that concerns you, identifying the specific behaviour and the effect it has on you as a member of the group by using 'I' statements. Using the formula *'when you do/say… I feel'* might be helpful.
- It might also be appropriate to state how you think the situation might be rectified.
- Alternatively, it might be appropriate to find out what impact the person thinks their lack of contribution has had on the group.
- It might be that there are particular circumstances that have affected their ability to make their contribution, which might or might not be divulged. Consider how you are going to empathize with the person or express your irritation if you consider it to be appropriate. For example, someone might say that they were unable to complete the work because their printer broke down and you feel that, although annoying, this was unavoidable.

Reflection on practice

- What do you like about being in a group?
- What annoys you about being in a group?
- To what extent do you feel you are able to communicate information that you had collected to other members of the group? Are there any other strategies that you might use to enhance your ability to give information?
- When working in a group, how have you provided feedback to at least one member of the group that you felt worked well?
- How successful are you in providing feedback to a group member who you felt did not do the work they had agreed to do?

- When you consider the group, do some people appear to feel excluded from the group? Do some people exclude themselves in the group? What impact does this have on you and how are you going to address it?

ACHIEVING CLOSURE IN PROFESSIONAL RELATIONSHIPS

Endings provide a variety of opportunities to develop our knowledge with regard to our relationships, our knowledge and our skills. There might be an opportunity to negotiate when the ending might occur or this might be predetermined: either way, those with whom you are working will need to be informed and reminded when this will take place. This is particularly important in practice placements for a number of reasons. It is highly likely that you have developed a good relationship with both patients and staff and so leaving unannounced will create varying levels of concern and possible anxiety (see Ch. 3).

A student once commented that she ended a placement without telling the patients with whom she had been working for 8 weeks that she was going. She did this because she did not want them to get upset. This is a good example of conscious incompetence (Howell 1982), in that the student had an awareness that leaving would have an effect on the patients, but she chose a strategy that would not relieve any anxieties that they might have about not seeing her; in fact, it might have heightened them. Interestingly, she did not comment on the effect that leaving the ward would have on her, until this was brought into her awareness through discussion.

Endings are likely to stimulate a sense of loss and the emergence of defensive feelings and behaviours that reflect those of loss and grief. This might include elements of denial, depression or acceptance. For example, a student might feel anxious and not ready to take on the responsibility of their first post as a registered nurse/midwife. As a consequence of this, they might delay applying for a job and preparation for interview until the very last minute, increasing the likelihood of being unsuccessful. This action could be considered as an unconscious defence leading to a self-fulfilling prophecy of not being good enough.

The practice of revisiting previous placements might be a defence against feeling loss and anxiety about moving on to another stage of development (see Appendix 2). Ideally, a state of acceptance of the sadness of leaving, with recognition that not all aspects of the experience might be missed, is desirable. Often there is a combination of excitement and anxiety at moving on to a new situation.

Achieving closure

You are in the last module of your course and have 3 weeks left of your placement. You have successfully completed all your assessments and have had a job interview, which you feel went well. Looking at your timetable, you notice that one of your study days has a reflection session scheduled. This will be your last session with your group.

The issues in this scenario provide ideas to help you make sense of and summarize your experiences throughout your course, and identify the transferability of the knowledge and skills that you have accomplished. There is also the opportunity to achieve satisfactory closure and prepare for the next stage of your development.

Specific principles

- Pre-registration nursing and midwifery education generally involves being part of a large cohort of students who receive lead lectures, the principles of which are then explored in greater detail in smaller seminar groups.

- The smaller groups might each consist of students studying for the same branch of nursing or it might be a mixed group. As well as being an aid to the development of practical skills, smaller groups can assist with the development of a more personal relationship with peers.

- Throughout training the group membership might change and this will have an effect on the group dynamics. Factors that might affect group members include patterns of poor attendance by some members, and when people leave or join the group.

- Changes in personal tutor or group/module leader might add to student anxieties since the 'secure base' from which to explore this learning experience has been disturbed (Bowlby 1988).

- Wherever possible, any changes in the group make-up should be made known without breaking confidentiality or with appropriate self-disclosure. For example, it is sufficient for a group member to say that they will be leaving the group without giving any further details.

- As an ending approaches, group members might begin to leave before the official leaving time occurs. This action not only discounts the value of the last episodes, as the person rushes to embrace the new experience, but also denies themselves and others the opportunity to give feedback and say goodbye. At an unconscious level, this strategy might serve to prevent the experience of sadness of leaving and/or fear of the future.

- Whether leaving a placement prior to commencing another or ending your education programme, experiences of regret might be evoked. Regret might be the result of having to leave just as you are beginning to understand the nature of the speciality and have become familiar with the team and the professional skills and activities.

Preparation of self

- What are you going to say to the patients you have been caring for with regard to the end of your placement?

- Which members of staff in particular need to be reminded that you will soon be leaving?

- Is there a session that is designed to help you reflect on your experiences?
- Are you going to attend the reflection session? If you decide that you are not, what do you imagine you might miss? If you decide to go, what would you like to achieve from the session?
- How do you feel about the fact that you are approaching the end of the module? It might be useful to make some private time available to explore this.
- Select a model of reflection that might help you record your experiences and reflections. Rolfe et al (2001) provide a critical selection from which to choose.
- Alternatively, you might wish to discuss this with a colleague to share thoughts and feelings. A number of authors recognize the positive value of undertaking reflection in a group (e.g. Bolton 2001, Hawkins & Shohet 2006, Sully et al 2008).
- If there is a staff nurse or midwife on your placement who has recently qualified, you might consider asking them how they felt when they were nearing registration.
- Consider speaking with your personal tutor, since they will be interested in helping you with this transition and they will also be preparing your reference and completing your personal file.
- Read what the literature has to say about the transition from student to registered nurse/midwife. This will help 'normalize' any concerns and anxieties that you have.

Putting the skills into practice

- Make a note of the things that need to be done when you leave the placement/course, for example completion of documentation. This might include such things as identifying a person to whom you wish to speak, submission dates for final assessments, or the gathering of books that need to be handed back to the library.
- Consult your journal or reflective notes before the reflection session so that you can make relevant personal contributions. This might add to your understanding of your current level of development.
- You might prefer to write about your experiences and the important moments in your course in the third person as this might help you to view it more objectively.
- Make appointments with those to whom you would like to speak for advice or in order to give appropriate feedback.
- At intervals throughout your final week, inform the patients in your care that you will be leaving the placement. This might be an opportunity to highlight your experience of caring for them and, if appropriate, the progress the patient has made during your time with them. Since the patients might have developed a strong bond with you, it is also important to reiterate the ability of those staff members who remain to care for them.
- An example of what to say as a leaving statement, is to identify what you will miss and what you are looking forward to (see Ch. 3 Leave-taking skills).

- Decide if there is anything special that you would like to do to mark the end of the course. It would be useful to investigate this and obtain relevant material should your group be interested in a group activity of some sort.

Reflection on practice

Referring to self-knowledge, Gibran (1991: 65) suggests that 'the treasure of your infinite depths would be revealed to your eyes'. One of the benefits of reflecting on an experience is to increase awareness and facilitate personal and professional development. If a period of time is not put aside to reflect at the end of a module of training or, indeed, at the end of a longer course, some of the significant contributors and contributions to your development (that might not be instantly obvious) can be missed. Gaining insight into your development through the exploration of concrete examples will help you discuss these at interview and have clearer ideas about your strength and areas for development. The following provide some strategies that you might use to capture those important episodes during your training. If you have been keeping a journal over the years, this will also facilitate the reflective process.

- What achievements would you like to celebrate as you approach this ending?
- What was it like when a new member joined your group?
- What was it like when you realized that someone had left the group?
- What do you imagine happened to them?
- How do you feel as you approach the end of this experience?
- What did you do as part of leaving each placement?
- How did others acknowledge that you were leaving the placement?
- What have you noticed about the different ways your group members are preparing for leaving the course? How can you help and support each other?
- Write a list of the people and aspects you are going to miss. Consider how you might keep memories of these, e.g. pictures, letters, contact details.
- Write a poem, story or letter that outlines your experience of the period of training.
- Draw a picture that symbolizes your experiences of being on the course.
- Draw a line to represent the beginning to the end of the course. Mark off significant highs and lows along the line and make notes about those times.
- Read through your journal, making a note of the date of the entries. This might help you make sense of the comments that you have made. For example, upon reading an entry that you made during the middle of your course you will be able to comment on the extent to which your level of knowledge, skills and confidence has developed. It might also be that your comments reflect events in your personal life or the nature of the speciality you were working in at the time.
- Looking back at the module or your course, is there anyone else you would like to give feedback or say goodbye to?

- Is there anyone you will be glad to leave behind? What have you learnt about yourself from this person?
- What have you learnt from doing any or all of the above activities?
- Write one sentence that sums up your experience of being on the course.

References

Baron, R., Kerr, N., 2003. Group Process, Group Decision, Group Action. Open University Press, Buckingham.

Belbin, M., 2003. Management Teams: Why They Succeed or Fail. Butterworth-Heinemann, Oxford.

Berne, E., 1966. Principles of Group Treatment. Shea Books, Menlo Park.

Bion, W., 1961. Experiences in Groups. Tavistock, London.

Bolton, G., 2001. Reflective Practice: Writing and Professional Development. Paul Chapman, London.

Bowlby, J., 1988. A Secure Base. Routledge, London.

Bradley, J., Edinberg, M., 1982. Communication in the Nursing Context. AC Crofts, New York.

Clarkson, P., 1993. Transactional Analysis Psychotherapy: An Integrated Approach. Routledge, London.

Gibran, K., 1991. The Prophet. Mandarin, London.

Hawkins, P., Shohet, R., 2006. Supervision in the Helping Professions, 3rd edn. Open University Press, Maidenhead.

Hayes, J., 2002. Interpersonal Skills at Work. Routledge, London.

Howell, W., 1982. The Empathic Communicator. Wadsworth, Pacific Grove.

Katzenbach, J.R., Smith, D.K., 1993. The Wisdom of Teams; Creating the High Performance Organization. Harvard Business School Press, Boston.

Larson, C., LaFasto, F., 1989. Teamwork. Sage, London.

Latane, B., Williams, K., Hoskins, S., 1979. Many hands make light work: the causes and consequences of social loafing. J. Pers. Soc. Psychol. 37, 822–832.

Napper, R., Newton, T., 2000. TACTICS. TA Resources, Ipswich.

Prosser, S., 2005. Effective People: Leadership and Organisation Development in Healthcare. Radcliffe, Oxford.

Rogers, C., 1961. On Becoming a Person. Constable, London.

Rolfe, G., Freshwater, D., Jasper, M., 2001. Critical Reflection for Nursing: A User's Guide. Palgrave, Hampshire.

Sully, P., Wandrag, M., Riddell, J., 2008. The use of reflective practice on masters programmes in interprofessional practice with survivors of intentional and unintentional violence. Reflective Practice 9 (2), 135–144.

Sundeen, S.J., Stuart, G., Rankin, E., Cohen, S.A., 1998. Nurse-Client Interaction: Implementing the Nursing Process, 7th edn. Mosby, St Louis.

Tuckman, B., 1965. Developmental sequences in small groups. Psychol. Bull. 63, 384–399.

Yalom, I., 1970. The Theory and Practice of Group Psychotherapy. Basic Books, New York.

Further reading

Glenny, G., Roaf, C., 2008. Multiprofessional Communication: Making systems work for children. Open University Press/McGraw Hill Education, Maidenhead.

10

Teaching skills

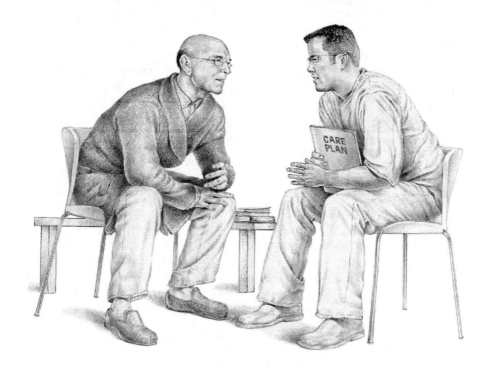

INTRODUCTION

Teaching is an integral part of nursing and midwifery practice (Kiger et al 2004) when working with patients, women who are pregnant or have become new mothers, families, clients, carers and colleagues. Benner (2001: 50) identifies teaching as part of the 'helping role' of the nurse. The Royal College of Midwives (2009) lists the wide variety of topics that are relevant to the midwife's role and thus identifies that teaching is integral to the midwife's role, e.g. in screening and health promotion, supporting breast-feeding, and in evidence-based practice.

Although this chapter addresses teaching patients and clients, the principles apply equally to teaching students and colleagues. The Nursing and Midwifery Council sets clear standards for the requirements to be met for the education and training of pre-registration nursing and midwifery students (Nursing and Midwifery Council 2004a,b): these requirements clearly state that registered practitioners have a responsibility also to support and teach the student nurses and midwives.

PRINCIPLES

There are a number of principles that apply to all situations when practitioners teach. Rogers (1961) argues that 'significant learning' changes us as people. Therefore in order to be effective in helping others to learn, practitioners need to base their teaching on an attitude of respect (Rogers 1983, 1961) for those in their care and for their circumstances.

Teaching to reduce dependence

Learning and teaching is a collaborative process. This is particularly significant in acute settings where patients are often dependent. Similarly women who are in labour, are dependent on the midwife's support and understanding of the process, a cooperative relationship being central to enabling them to respond appropriately when advised by the practitioner. In such settings, it is important to use teaching to promote their independence. Practitioners' encouragement that 'involves (their) relinquishing power and control over them, and which instead facilitates their empowerment' (Latter 1998: 13), enables them to gain knowledge and skills that can free them from dependence on the nurse or midwife.

By demonstrating empathetic recognition of the patient's or woman's concerns about the topic or process to be taught, the practitioner lays the foundation for trust. Trust is an essential component of the helping relationship (Sundeen et al 1998, Rogers 1957) through which those in our care can express their thoughts and feelings about what they are learning.

Adult learning

Arguably, the majority of people who midwives and nurses teach are adults, in that they are most likely to be 16 years of age or older. Knowles et al (2005: 199) state that 'Adults tend to be motivated towards learning that helps them solve problems in their lives or results in internal payoffs'. Adults learn best therefore when they recognize that they need to learn, e.g. a new skill as a pre-registration student or a mother's different way of managing her infant feeding when her new baby doesn't seem to settle. Adults are thus also more likely to be self motivated.

Frequently, those in our care who need to understand their changed health situations or their new status such as being parents, are facing major life transitions. It is for this reason that practitioners need always to remember their responsibilities to approach those they are teaching with respect and empathy, recognizing that anxiety and intense emotions can interfere with peoples' capacities to learn and thus acquire new skills and attitudes to deal with their new situations.

It is also important to recognize that people have individual learning styles (Knowles et al 2005, Dean & Kenworthy 2000). Therefore it is essential that the specific needs and circumstances of patients, women, their carers and/or loved ones are taken into account when planning, implementing and evaluating teaching, to ensure that these issues are accommodated.

Preparation for teaching

The practitioner must be well-informed about the topic to be addressed. The session should be prepared in advance, whether it is a formal or informal session, and even if time is short. There should be clear aims and learning outcomes for the session. The practitioner needs to be clear about exactly what the person needs to know and how it will be taught. The subject and focus of the session therefore needs to be decided **in collaboration** with the client. Practitioners also need to be aware that clients, while recognizing that they *do* need to learn, might not know the **essential components** of what they are setting out to learn.

Teaching notes should be written to ensure that information is up-to-date and nothing essential is omitted. Cards are useful when working on the practice area, as they are easily kept in pockets or equipment bags. Time must be set aside for the teaching and the venue where the teaching takes place has to be prepared to ensure as far as possible that it is quiet, that as little as possible is likely to be overheard, and there are no interruptions. This allows for the client to ask questions and express concerns. Set any tables and chairs in a manner that does not form a barrier between the practitioner and the client.

Any apparatus used, such as blood-monitoring equipment or an overhead projector, must be checked to ensure it is functioning correctly and any written information must be up-to-date and correct. In order to help build a collaborative working relationship, it is important for us to introduce ourselves and invite the patients, women and clients to use our preferred name. Introduce the topic and explain the reasons why it is important that they are well-informed about it. It is important to start with what they understand and/or what skills they can already perform. Thus clarification of their knowledge and skills is crucial before introducing new information and/or techniques to them.

Note: In all circumstances, practitioners should ensure that they are competent to teach the topic, process or practical skill. **Students should always be supervised**, unless formally deemed competent by a qualified practitioner to teach unsupervised. The qualified practitioner is accountable, but the student is responsible for agreeing that they are able to undertake the task.

Teaching methods

The method of teaching must be appropriate for the topic, e.g. practical skills must be demonstrated and not just discussed. Clients should also be able to practise the skills under the supervision of the practitioner. Information and skills should be broken down into their component parts and given in a logical sequence. The practitioner should choose language that is appropriate for the client's understanding. Jargon and technical terms should be avoided and cue cards or an interpreter should be used if necessary.

Body language should demonstrate respect; it is usually inappropriate to stand over a client when teaching. It is better to be at the same level as them and be aware of physical proximity, so as not to be perceived as intimidating. Most clients are likely to have had experience of being taught, some of which may not have been pleasant. Being taught could elicit discomfiting memories (see Ch. 1).

Checking understanding

The practitioner must check the client's understanding at regular intervals and correct it if necessary. Wherever possible, written information for the client to refer to afterwards should be given. If appropriate, this should include contact details of the ward and/or service and support organizations. The practitioner should continually evaluate the teaching, checking the client's understanding by asking them to explain exactly what they understand from the session. This can be done through careful questioning (see Ch. 5).

Learning from experience

When we teach patients we include them in the process, thereby offering them an experience that is relevant to their learning needs. Steinaker & Bell (1979) describe the processes of learning from experience as follows (Nicklin 2000: 21):

- **Exposure level** – where the learner is exposed to an experience and conscious that this is so
- **Participation level** – where the learner decides to be actively involved in the process of learning from the experience
- **Identification level** – where the learner identifies with the experience and sees its relevance to them, both emotionally and intellectually

- **Internalization level** – where the new learning becomes an integral part of the learner's personal knowledge and understanding, and their behaviour changes as a result
- **Dissemination level** – where the learner passes the experiential learning on to others.

TEACHING PEOPLE IN OUR CARE

Much of what we teach clients has to do with what is likely to occur, i.e. a process, such as being discharged, rather than solely a topic, such as details about their condition. We therefore need to recognize the differences in helping those in our care to understand the *processes* they are likely to experience as well as *specific topics*.

Teaching a patient how to take medication

A middle-aged patient has asked you to explain why it is so important that she remembers to take her medication for hypertension.

Some issues raised by this scenario:
- How well you know the person in your care
- Your knowledge of the importance of medication for hypertension
- Whether you should seek help from a more experienced practitioner or the pharmacist.

Preparation of self

- What do you know about your client, their individual circumstances (not solely their diagnosis and treatment) and how these relate to the teaching of this topic? Note their age, gender and culture so you can choose appropriate language and examples.
- Clarify exactly what your client needs to learn.
- What literature or information do you need on the subject?
- Ensure that all the information you have is correct and up-to-date.
- Write brief aims and learning outcomes for the teaching session.
- Write notes to ensure the important points are not omitted. Collect together any equipment you will be using.
- Ensure that you have any written information you think the client might find useful to keep, including contact and support group details.

Environment

- The environment should be private and as quiet as possible, preferably where the teaching cannot be overheard and away from distractions.

- Allow enough time for the session.
- It may be appropriate to involve a family member in the teaching if the person would like this and you are confident that this is in their best interests.

Putting the skills into practice

- Introduce the topic by explaining clearly the purpose of the teaching, e.g. to ensure that they understand the importance of taking their medication regularly.
- Ask the client what they know about their condition and their medication.
- Clarify with the client exactly what you understand it is important for them to know, i.e. the learning outcomes you have prepared.
- Explain the topic in a logical sequence, linking it to the client's own stated knowledge.
- Ensure you have included all the essential information.
- Help the client to understand by making the information relevant to their own circumstances. For example, ask them about their daily routine so that the times they are most likely to remember to take their medication can be identified.
- Observe throughout the session for verbal and non-verbal signs of their level of understanding.
- At regular intervals, ask the client to repeat to you what they understand of what you have explained and clarify any misunderstandings.
- Evaluate the session at the end by asking the person to explain to you, exactly what they have understood. Reinforce any omitted points and correct any misunderstandings.
- Reinforce learning by giving the client written information on the topic, with contact details if appropriate.

Reflection on practice

Think about a situation from your practice when you taught a patient, woman or client about a topic.

- How successful were you in your preparation for the teaching session?
- What aspects of the environment were appropriate? If the environment was not ideal, what did you do to ensure as much privacy and quiet for the person as possible?
- How did you feel before, during and after your teaching session?
- How do you think these feelings might have influenced how you taught, the language you used and how the person experienced the learning process?
- How successful were you in encouraging them to learn in partnership with you?

- What insights did you gain when you evaluated their learning at the end of the session? How will this help you develop your teaching skills further?

Explaining the process for follow-up care for a newborn baby

You have attended Mrs Richards during her labour and delivery. She is ready to be discharged with specialist follow-up care for her baby, in the community. She has asked you to explain what will happen.

Some issues raised by this scenario:

- The importance of ensuring the coordination of services for support in the community by clear communication with the interprofessional team involved with her care (see Ch. 6).
- Mrs Richards needs to understand that discharge from hospital to the community is a process. This means that a team, rather than just one person, is likely to be involved in her baby's care in the community.

Preparation of self

- What do you know about the person in your care, her individual circumstances and those of her baby (not solely the details of the delivery, the reason for the community follow-up and relevant diagnosis and treatment). How are these related to teaching her about her baby's care in the community? Note her age and culture so you can choose appropriate language and examples.
- Clarify exactly what Mrs Richards needs to learn about her baby's follow-up care in the community.
- What literature and information do you need on the subject?
- Ensure that all the information you have is correct and up-to-date.
- Write brief aims and learning outcomes for the teaching session.
- Write notes to ensure the important points are not omitted. Collect together any equipment you will be using.
- Ensure that you have any written information that you think Mrs Richards might find useful to keep, including contact and support group details, e.g. groups for new mothers.

Environment

- The environment should be private and as quiet as possible, preferably where the teaching cannot be overheard and without interruptions and distractions.
- Allow enough time for the teaching session, or divide it into separate parts for different times.

- It may be appropriate to involve Mrs Richards' partner or close friend if she would like this, and you are confident that she regards this as being in her and her/their baby's best interests.

Putting the skills into practice

- Introduce the topic by explaining clearly the purpose of the teaching, e.g. to ensure that Mrs Richards understands the sequence of events leading up to and after discharge from hospital.
- Ask her what she knows about the plans for her baby's care in the community.
- Clarify with her exactly what you understand is important for her to know, i.e. the learning outcomes you have prepared.
- Explain the discharge process in a logical sequence, linking it to Mrs Richards' own stated knowledge.
- Observe throughout the session for verbal and non-verbal signs of her level of understanding.
- Ensure you have included all the essential information, e.g. which community paediatrician and midwifery team will be providing the follow-up care.
- Help her to understand by making the information relevant to her own circumstances.
- At regular intervals, ask Mrs Richards to repeat to you what she understands you to have informed her about and clarify any misunderstandings.
- Evaluate the session at the end by asking Mrs Richards to explain to you exactly what she has understood. Reinforce any omitted points and correct any misunderstandings.
- Reinforce her learning by providing written information on the services she will receive in the community, with contact details as appropriate.

Reflection on practice

Think about a situation from your practice when you have had to teach a woman, patient, client or relative (such as a parent) about the process of being referred on to other members of the interprofessional healthcare team.

- How successful were you in your preparation for the teaching session?
- How much were you able to involve the interprofessional team concerned with the person's care in the preparation for this session?
- What aspects of the environment where you taught were appropriate? If the environment was not ideal, what did you do to ensure as much privacy and quiet for the client as possible?
- How successful were you in encouraging your client to learn in partnership with you?
- How did you feel before, during and after your teaching session?

- How do you think these feelings might have influenced how you taught, the language you used and how your client experienced the learning process?
- After evaluating their learning with the client, what did you learn that will help you develop further your teaching skills?

TEACHING A PRACTICAL SKILL

Learning and teaching practical skills are integral to nursing and midwifery practice (Neary 2000). As professional practitioners we often need to teach those in our care new practical skills such as mixing their babies' feeds or managing their stomas. Learning new practical skills can be daunting for many people, especially when we appear to demonstrate them with ease. People are able to take control of their healthcare needs if they are able to learn the necessary practical skills, such as giving themselves injections or ensuring that they sterilize their babies' bottles correctly. Taking on these responsibilities for themselves can give them a sense of accomplishment and empowerment (see also Ch. 5).

Teaching a pregnant woman to monitor her blood sugar levels

Under the supervision of her mentor, a student is asked to teach a woman with gestational diabetes how to monitor her blood sugar levels.

Some issues raised by this scenario:

- The need for supervision and knowledge of the technique and standard precautions
- The need to break a complex skill into manageable steps.

Preparation of self

- What do you know about the person in your care, their individual circumstances (not solely the duration of their pregnancy or their diagnosis and treatment) and how these relate to the teaching of this topic?

  Note: Remember their age, gender and culture so you can choose appropriate language and examples.
- Clarify with them exactly what they need to learn.
- What literature or information do you need on the subject? Ensure that all the information you have is correct and up-to-date.
- Write brief aims and learning outcomes for the teaching session and notes to ensure the important points are not omitted.
- Collect together any equipment you will be using.
- Ensure that you have any written information that you think the client might find useful to keep, including contact and support group details.

- Prepare all the equipment needed for the demonstration, e.g. gloves, blood glucose meter, finger-pricking device or lancet, gauze swab or cotton ball (according to policy), blood glucose testing strips (Nicol et al 2008: 36).
- Ensure that you are observing universal precautions.
- Ensure that a qualified member of staff observes your practice of the skill and considers that you are competent to teach it.
- Practise the skill to ensure you are proficient in doing it yourself and you feel confident to teach it.
- Then break it down into component parts and prepare what you need to say during each stage of the demonstration. These steps may need to be taught on separate occasions, e.g. pricking the finger and obtaining a good blood sample on one occasion and using the glucose meter on another occasion.
- Ensure your own proficiency in the skill as well as breaking it down into steps and explaining them, as you demonstrate each step.

Environment

- The environment should be quiet.
- Set aside enough time for the woman to accomplish the skill. It is wise to be generous with the time rather than hurry her while she is practising the skill.
- Ensure there is enough equipment for you to demonstrate more than once if necessary and for the woman to practise with.
- On completion, tidy the environment and put all equipment away.
- Ensure that any disposable equipment is discarded appropriately, e.g. disposing of the lance in a sharps bin.

Putting the skills into practice

- Ensure you have all the equipment necessary for the demonstration.
- Ensure the woman is positioned comfortably and can see clearly what you are demonstrating.
- Establish whether she is right- or left-handed.
- Ensure you are observing universal precautions throughout the demonstration.
- Explain to the woman the skill you are about to teach them and the reasons.
- Explain clearly all the equipment and its relevance.
- Demonstrate the complete skill.
- Then demonstrate the first part of the skill, explaining what you are doing throughout the process, e.g. how to hold a lancet.
- Observe for verbal and non-verbal signs of her level of understanding.
- Now, encourage the woman to try out the first part of the skill with you. Do not move on to the second part of the skill until this is firmly understood.

This may well take several sessions with a complex skill such as blood glucose monitoring. The woman can gradually assume more responsibility for the parts of the skill as she accomplishes each part.

- Explain clearly the process as she practises each component part and learns to link them together.
- Encourage her to ask questions, clarify points and explain any difficulties she might be encountering.
- Allow time for her to keep practising the skill until both you and she are sure she is competent.
- An accurate demonstration by the woman is a sound means of evaluating your teaching session.
- Ensure that she is supervised until you both feel confident that she can do it alone.
- Throughout the process offer the woman positive feedback and encouragement, helping her to use her strengths to accomplish those aspects of the skill she might be finding more difficult.

Reflection on practice

Think about a situation from your practice when you have been involved in teaching a woman or client a practical skill.

- How successful were you in your preparation for the teaching and demonstration of the skill?
- What aspects of the environment where you taught were appropriate?
- If the environment was not ideal, what did you do to ensure as much privacy and quiet for your client as possible?
- How did you feel before, during and after your teaching session?
- How do you think these feelings might have influenced how you taught, the language you used and how the woman experienced the learning process?
- After evaluating the patient's learning and receiving feedback from your supervisor, what did you learn that will help you develop your teaching skills further?

References

Benner, P.E., 2001. From Novice to Expert. Excellence and Power in Clinical Nursing Practice. Commemorative edn. Addison-Wesley, Menlo Park.

Dean, J., Kenworthy, N., 2000. The principles of learning. In: Nicklin, P.J., Kenworthy, N. (Eds.), Teaching and Assessing in Nursing Practice: An Experiential Approach, 3rd edn. Baillière Tindall, London, pp. 45–67.

Kiger, A.M., Coutts, L.C., Hardy, L.K., 2004. Teaching for Health, 3rd edn. Elsevier, Edinburgh.

Knowles, M.S., Holton III, E.F., Swanson, R.A., 2005. The Adult Learner, 6th edn. Elsevier, Amsterdam.

Latter, S., 1998. Health promotion in the acute setting: the case for empowering nurses. In: Kendall, S. (Ed.), Health and Empowerment: Research and Practice. Arnold, London, pp. 11–37.

Neary, M., 2000. Teaching, Assessing and Evaluation for Clinical Competence. A Practical Guide for Practitioners and Teachers. Stanley Thorne, Cheltenham.

Nicklin, P.J., 2000. Quality in teaching practice. In: Nicklin, P.J., Kenworthy, N. (Eds.), Teaching and Assessing in Nursing Practice: An Experiential Approach, 3rd edn. Baillière Tindall, London.

Nicol, M., Bavin, C., Cronin, P., Rawlings-Anderson, K., 2008. Essential Nursing Skills, 3rd edn. Mosby, Edinburgh.

Nursing and Midwifery Council, 2004a. Standards of Proficiency for Pre-Registration Nursing Education. Online. Available at: www.nmc-uk.org/aDisplayDocument. aspx?documentID=328 (accessed 2 August 2009).

Nursing and Midwifery Council, 2004b. Standards of proficiency for pre-registration midwifery education. Online. Available at: www.nmc-uk.org/aArticle.aspx?ArticleID=2867 (accessed 2 August 2009).

Rogers, C., 1957. The necessary and sufficient conditions of therapeutic personality change. J. Consult. Psychol. 21, 95–103.

Rogers, C., 1961. On Becoming a Person. Constable, London.

Rogers, C., 1983. Freedom to Learn for the 80s. Merrill, Columbus.

Royal College of Midwives, website. Online. Available at: www.rcm.org.uk/by-subject (accessed 25 April 2009).

Steinaker, N., Bell, R., 1979. The Experiential Taxonomy: a New Approach to Teaching and Learning. Academic Press, New York.

Sundeen, S.J., Stuart, G.W., Rankin, E.A.D., Cohen, S.A., 1998. Nurse-client Interaction: Implementing the Nursing Process, 7th edn. Mosby, St Louis.

Further reading
Cadwell, K., Turner-Maffei, C., 2009. Continuity of Care in Breastfeeding: Best Practices in the Maternity Setting. Jones and Bartlett, London.

Johnson, R., Taylor, W., 2004. Skills for Midwifery Practice. Churchill Livingstone, London.

Nolan, M.L., Foster, J., 2005. Birth and Parenting Skills – New Directions in Antenatal Education. Elsevier Churchill Livingstone, London.

Bibliography

Armstrong, D., 2005. Organization in the Mind. Karnac, London.

Barber, P., 2001. Respect. Nurs. Times 97, 23–25.

Becker, C., 1992. Living and Relating. Sage, London.

Belbin, R.M., 1996. Team Roles at Work. Butterworth Heinemann, Oxford.

Bingler, R., 2001. Communicating genetic test results to the family: a six step skills-building strategy. Fam. Community Health 24, 13–26.

Bor, R., Watts, M., 1993. Talking to patients about sexual matters. Br. J. Nurs. 2, 657–661.

Bowlby, J., 1988. A Secure Base. Clinical Applications of Attachment Theory. Tavistock/Routledge, London.

Buckman, R., 2001. Communication skills in palliative care: a practical guide. Neurol. Clin. 19, 989–1004.

Burstow, B., 1992. Radical Feminist Therapy. Working in the Context of Violence. Sage, London.

Cadwell, K., Turner-Maffei, C., 2009. Continuity of Care in Breastfeeding: Best Practices in the Maternity Setting. Jones and Bartlett, London.

Casement, P., 1985. On Learning from the Patient. Routledge, London.

Casement, P., 1990. Further Learning from the Patient. The Analytic Space and Process. Routledge, London.

Chapey, R., 2001. Language Intervention Strategies in Aphasia and Related Neurogenic Communication Disorders, 4th edn. Lippincott Williams and Wilkins, Philadelphia.

Chauhan, G., Long, A., 2000. Communication is the essence of nursing care 1: breaking bad news. Br. J. Nurs. 9, 931–938.

Chauhan, G., Long, A., 2000. Communication is the essence of nursing care 2: breaking bad news. Br. J. Nurs. 9, 979–984.

Crouch, S., 1999. Sexual health 1: sexuality and nurses' role in sexual health. Br. J. Nurs. 8, 601–606.

Crouch, S., 1999. Sexual health 2: an overt approach to sexual health education. Br. J. Nurs. 8, 669–675.

Doyal, L., 2001. Sex, gender and health: the need for a new approach. Br. Med. J. 323 (7320), 1061–1063.

Dean, J., Kenworthy, N., 2000. The principles of learning. In: Nicklin, P.J., Kenworthy, N. (Eds.), Teaching and Assessing in Nursing Practice: An Experiential Approach, 3rd edn. Baillière Tindall, London, pp. 45–67.

Dunhill, A., Elliott, B., Shaw, A. (Eds.), 2009. Effective Communication with Children and Young People, their Families and Carers. Learning Matters, Exeter.

Evans, D., 2000. Speaking of sex: the need to dispel myths and overcome fears. Br. J. Nurs. 9, 650–655.

Freshwater, D., 2002. Therapeutic Nursing. Sage, London.

Glenny, G., Roaf, C., 2008. Multiprofessional Communication: Making systems work for children. Open University Press/McGraw Hill Education, Maidenhead.

Golman, D., 1998. Working with Emotional Intelligence. Bloomsbury, London.

Grasha, A.F., 1995. Practical Applications of Psychology, 4th edn. HarperCollins, New York.

Hackman, J., 1986. The design of work teams. In: Lorsch, J. (Ed.), Handbook of Organizational Behaviour. Prentice Hall, New Jersey.

Hare, A., 1982. Creativity in Small Groups. Sage, Beverley Hills.

Hawkins, P., Shohet, R., 2006. Supervision in the Helping Professions. Open University Press, Maidenhead.

Hinshelwood, R.D., Skogstad, W., (Eds.), 2000. Observing Organisations. Routledge, London.

Hoban, V., 2003. How to handle a handover. Nurs. Times 99, 54–55.

Huffington, C., Armstrong, D., Halton, H., Hoyle, L., Pooley, J., 2004. Working below the surface. Karnac, London.

Hughes, L., Pengelly, P., 1997. Staff Supervision in a Turbulent Environment: Managing Process and Task in Front-line Services. Jessica Kingsley, London.

Janis, I., 1982. Groupthink. Houghton Mifflin, Boston.

Jarvis, P., Holford, J., Griffin, C., 2003. The Theory and Practice of Learning, 2nd edn. Kogan Page, London.

Johns, C., Freshwater, D., 2005. Transforming Nursing through Reflective Practice. Blackwell, Oxford.

Johnson, R., Taylor, W., 2004. Skills for Midwifery Practice. Churchill Livingstone, London.

Kiger, A.M., Coutts, L.C., Hardy, L.K., 2004. Teaching for Health, 3rd edn. Elsevier, Edinburgh.

Knowles, M.S., Holton III, E.F., Swanson, R.A., 2005. The Adult Learner, 6th edn. Elsevier, Amsterdam.

Malan, D.H., 1995. Individual Psychotherapy and the Science of Psychodynamics. 2nd edn. Hodder Arnold, London.

McGee, P., 1994. The concept of respect in nursing. Br. J. Nurs. 3, 681–684.

Milner, P., Carolin, B., 1999. Time to Listen to Children: Personal and Professional Communication. Routledge, London.

Nelson-Jones, R., 2008. Basic Counselling Skills, 2nd edn. Sage, London.

Nelson-Jones, R., 2006. Human Relationship Skills, 4th edn. Routledge, London.

Nelson-Jones, R., 2001. Theory and Practice of Counselling and Therapy, 3rd edn. Sage, London.

Nicklin, P.J., Kenworthy, N. (Eds.), 2000. Teaching and Assessing in Nursing Practice: An Experiential Approach. Baillière Tindall, London.

Nicol, M., Bavin, C., Bedford-Turner, S., Cronin, P., Rawlings-Anderson, K., 2008. Essential Nursing Skills, 3rd edn. Mosby, Edinburgh.

Nolan, M.L., Foster, J., 2005. Birth and Parenting Skills – New Directions in Antenatal Education. Elsevier Churchill Livingstone, London.

Obholzer, A., Roberts, V.Z. (Eds.), 1994. The Unconscious at Work: Individual and Organizational Stress in the Human Services. Routledge, London.

Palmer, S., McMahon, G., 1997. Handbook of Counselling, 2nd edn. Routledge/British Association for Counselling, London.

Pederson, P., 1995. The Five Stages of Culture Shock. Greenwood Press, London.

Petrie, P., 1997. Communicating with Children and Adults: Interpersonal Skills for Early Years and Playwork. Edward Arnold, London.

Quill, T., 2000. Initiating end-of-life discussions with seriously ill patients: addressing the "elephant in the room". J. Am. Med. Assoc. 284, 2502–2507.

Reid, M., Hammersley, R., 2000. Communicating Successfully in Groups. Routledge, London.

Reynolds, W., Scott, B., 1999. Empathy: a crucial component of the helping relationship. J Psychiatr. Ment. Health. Nurs. 6, 363–370.

Richardson, J., Burnard, P., 1994. Talking with children: some basic counselling skills. Prof. Care Mother Child May, 111–114.

Royal College of Nursing, 2002. Caring for Children. RCN, London.

Saunders, P., 1994. First Steps in Counselling. PCCS Books, Manchester.

Scheick, D., 2002. Mastering group leadership: an active learning experience. J. PsychoSoc. Nurs. 40, 30–39.

Schön, D.A., 1991. The Reflective Practitioner: How Professionals Think in Action. Basic Books, London.

Scrutton, S., 1999. Counselling Older People. Arnold, London.

Seiser, L., Wastell, C., 2002. Interventions and Techniques. Open University Press, Buckingham.

Spector, R., 2008. Cultural Diversity in Health and Illness. Pearson, Warwickshire.

Stevenson, C., Grieves, M., Stein-Parbury, J., 2004. Patient and Person. Elsevier Churchill Livingstone, Edinburgh.

Vreede, V., 2001. Life and loss counselling. Psychother. J. 12, 7–9.

Winnicott, D.W., 1986. Home is Where We Start From. Penguin, Harmondsworth.

Wright, H., 1989. Groupwork: Perspectives and Practice. Scutari Press, London.

Wykes, T., (Ed.), 1994. Violence and Health Care Professionals. Chapman & Hall, London.

Appendix 1 – Glossary

Boundaries

Boundaries clarify the extent and limits of professional practice. They provide containment, physical and psychological safety for both practitioners and those with whom they work, and ensure that unnecessary intrusions are avoided (see Pilette et al 1995).

'Cared for'

When a practitioner pays attention to (and addresses as much as is appropriate) the psychological and physical needs of patients, they are more likely to feel cared for. Being 'cared for' involves a demonstration of compassion and a concern for the wellbeing of the patient and may also include the use of advanced empathy. Patients may feel the practitioner warmth toward them.

Congruence/incongruence

'...a matching of experience, awareness and communication' (Rogers 1967: 339). For example, a patient asks the practitioner or midwife if they could spare some time to talk to them about their medication. The practitioner is aware of the patient's need, says 'Yes' and proceeds to sit and talk with the patient, in an attentive manner. An example of incongruence would be where the practitioner said 'Yes' but did not demonstrate that they were available to the patient by sitting and paying attention. Occasionally in practice, there may be times when the internal experience and awareness are not able to be communicated, e.g. in the case of an ethical dilemma. Since practitioner and midwives belong to professions, they may be involved in treatments and care that are incongruent practice with their personal values. This may result in conflict regarding other roles they have in society, with their own values or with the values of those for whom they are caring and/or with whom they are working (see Nelson-Jones 2006, 2001).

Containment

Containment is the sense of psychological safety offered by the skilful use of therapeutic boundaries which help the patient feel supported and safe. It is also important for practitioners to manage their professional boundaries so that they can remain task-focused (Obholzer & Roberts 1994) and not become overwhelmed by the demands of their role.

Countertransference

This is unconsciously responding in the here-and-now to another person's transference, e.g. the patient's transference to the practitioner on whom they are dependent, rather than the practitioner responding to what the patient actually needs in that specific moment. In this way, the practitioner is fulfilling the unconscious role in which the patient or client sees them, i.e. practitioner act out the countertransference relationship, which fulfils the patient's expectations from the past (see Jacobs 2004).

Ego state model

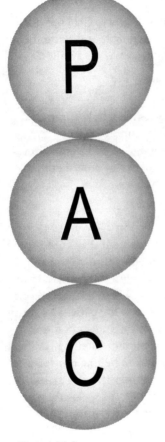

Parent Ego State

Thoughts, feelings and behaviours copied from parent or parent figures. When a parent ego state is drawn with a line down the middle and divided into Controlling (CP), and Nurturing Parent (NP), this represents the functional model. This is because it symbolizes how we function in the world. CP represents those aspects of discipline and control we have experienced and currently use. NP reflects our experience of, and ability to show, care and concern for ourselves and others.

Adult Ego State

Thoughts, feelings and behaviours related to here-and-now perceptions.

Child Ego State

Thoughts, feelings and behaviours related to childhood perceptions. When the Child ego state is drawn with a line down the middle and divided into Adapted Child (AC) and Free Child (FC), this also represents the functional model. AC represents behaviour that is adapted, for example, in order to seek approval. FC reflects our uncensored abilities, for example, in being spontaneous, creative and playful.

Figure A1.1

Gallows laugh

This is a laugh that accompanies a statement or experience that is unpleasant. The laugh is incongruent with what is happening at the time.

Hook or gimmick

In communication, the 'hook' or the 'gimmick' is the part of an individual that is vulnerable and leads them to follow a certain course of action at the invitation of another. While this is enacted at an unconscious level, the individual feels drawn to do or say something, even although the outcome may not be desirable. The process and the outcome feels familiar. In transactional analysis, this is part of the sequence in a game (see Berne 1975).

Paralinguistics

This is the term used to describe the tone, timbre and intonation that accompanies speech. Paralinguistics enable individuals to perceive people's moods or intentions, even if they cannot see them, such as when speaking on the telephone.

Secure base/environment

Child development studies identify how the infant explores its surroundings. A key feature of this exploration is the frequent returning to the central figure with whom they are familiar and feel safe and secure. This is generally a parent or guardian (see Ainsworth et al 1978). A secure base may be either physical or psychological (or both): a room, building or person, e.g. where the individual feels safe enough to do what needs to be done or indeed do nothing at all. For patients, this may be the return to the ward and familiar faces following treatment in the physiotherapy department, which they may have experienced as stressful.

Self-disclosure

This is an activity which may be verbal or non-verbal, intentional or unintentional and involves revealing something personal, e.g. how you are feeling. Appropriate self-disclosure is an important part of human relationships. However, practice varies across gender, cultures and context. The boundaries surrounding self-disclosure need to be considered.

Self-fulfilling prophecy

This occurs when actions are taken (either consciously or unconsciously) that increase the likelihood of an imagined outcome becoming a reality. For example, students may fear not being able to complete an assignment because they do not think they know enough. Time may be spent procrastinating and worrying about the outcome of not producing their assignment, instead of getting on with the work. The result may be that the work is not done as well as it could have been and the students are left feeling as they had originally predicted.

Silence

Being quiet and still with those in distress demonstrates the capacity to 'be with' (Benner 2001: 50) them or alongside them. Sometimes it demands self-discipline not to fill in the space left by the silence. It also allows the opportunity for reflection and disclosure if this is what is needed.

Therapeutic relationship

This is the relationship between the professional practitioner and the patient/client, the focus of which is the benefit of the patient/client. The practitioner uses their skills in partnership, wherever possible, with the patient/client. The core conditions of all therapeutic relationships (Rogers 1957) form the foundation of any effective professional practitioner–client relationship.

Transactions

Berne (1961) described a transaction as a unit of social intercourse. A transaction stimulus (S) from one person is followed by a transaction response (R) from the other person. There are a number of types of transactions, but three will be used to illustrate the concept. These are complementary, crossed and ulterior. The ego state model is used to analyse transactions (see also Tilney 1998).

Complementary transaction
The ego state that replies is the one that was addressed. This facilitates the continuance of communication.

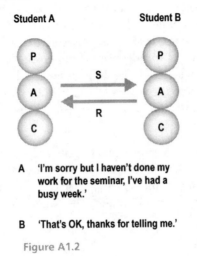

A	'I'm sorry but I haven't done my work for the seminar, I've had a busy week.'
B	'That's OK, thanks for telling me.'

Figure A1.2

Crossed transaction
This leads to a breakdown in communication, since the ego state that is addressed is not the one that replies. Communication can only resume if one or both change ego states.

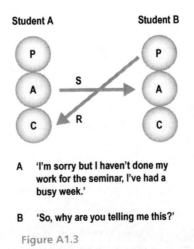

A	'I'm sorry but I haven't done my work for the seminar, I've had a busy week.'
B	'So, why are you telling me this?'

Figure A1.3

Ulterior transaction

This type of transaction occurs when two messages are sent simultaneously, one at the social level and the other at the psychological level. This is represented in the diagram by a broken line and 'p'. The outcome is always determined at the psychological level (see Stewart 2007 for a more in-depth discussion).

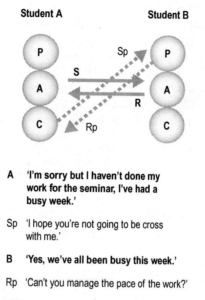

A   'I'm sorry but I haven't done my work for the seminar, I've had a busy week.'

Sp 'I hope you're not going to be cross with me.'

B   'Yes, we've all been busy this week.'

Rp 'Can't you manage the pace of the work?'

Figure A1.4

Transference

Transference is unconsciously relating in the here-and-now to another person, as if they were a different, usually emotionally significant, person from their past (see Jacobs 2004, Nelson-Jones 2001).

Triangle of insight

The triangle of insight enables the practitioner and/or the patient to interpret what the patient might be experiencing, by linking the patient's behaviour in relation to the practitioner in the here-and-now with the patient's behaviour in the present but with other people, which in turn can be linked to the patient's/client's experiences as a child with primary carers (see Jacobs 2004: 139).

References

Ainsworth, M., Blehar, M., Waters, E., Wilson, K.B.S., 2009. Patterns of Attachment: A Psychological Study of the Strange Situation. Erlbaum, New Jersey.

Benner, P., 2001. From Novice to Expert. Excellence and Power in Clinical Nursing Practice. Prentice Hall, New Jersey.

Berne, E., 1961. Transactional Analysis in Psychotherapy. Grove Press, New York.

Berne, E., 1975. What Do You Say After You Say Hello? Corgi, London.

Jacobs, M., 2004. Psychodynamic Counselling in Action, 3rd edn. Sage, London.

Nelson-Jones, R., 2001. Theory and Practice of Counselling and Therapy, 3rd edn. Sage, London.

Nelson-Jones, R., 2006. Human Relationship Skills, 4th edn. Routledge, London.

Obholzer, A., Roberts, V.Z., 1994. The Unconscious at Work: Individual and Organizational Stress in the Human Services. Routledge, London.

Pilette, P.C., Berck, C.B., Achber, L.C., 1995. Therapeutic management of helping boundaries. J. Psychosoc. Nurs. 33 (1), 40–47.

Rogers, C., 1957. The necessary and sufficient conditions of therapeutic personality change. J. Consult Psychol. 21, 95–103.

Rogers, C., 1967. On Becoming a Person. Constable, London.

Stewart, I., 2007. Transactional Analysis Counselling in Action, 3rd edn. Sage, London.

Tilney, T., 1998. Dictionary of Transactional Analysis. Whurr, London.

Appendix 2 – Some unconscious ego defences

Adapted from Gross, R., 2005. *Psychology: The Science of Mind and Behaviour*, 5th edn. Hodder and Stoughton Educational, London.

Name of defence	Description
Repression	Forcing a threatening or distressing memory, feeling or wish out of consciousness and making it unconscious
Displacement	Transferring our feelings from their true target on to a harmless, substitute target ('kicking the cat' instead of the person who has caused the upset)
Denial	Failing or refusing to acknowledge or perceive some aspect of reality
Rationalization	Finding an acceptable excuse (a 'cover story' that can sound very plausible) for some really quite unacceptable behaviour or situation
Reaction-formation	Consciously feeling or thinking the opposite of your true (unconscious) feelings or thoughts
Sublimation	A form of displacement in which a (socially positive) substitute activity is found for expressing some unacceptable impulse
Identification	Incorporating or introjecting another person into one's own personality – making him or her part of oneself
Projection	Displacing your own unacceptable feelings or characteristics on to someone else
Regression	Reverting to behaviour characteristics of an earlier stage of development
Isolation	Separating contradictory thoughts or feelings into 'logic-tight' compartments

Appendix 3 – Explaining obstetric terminology in an emergency

Note: The drawings are for illustration of positions being explained. It is crucial that in practice, women are covered with modesty sheets to preserve their dignity. Drawings courtesy of Martin Laurence.
Adapted from M. Baron (2009) London: *Teaching Notes*.

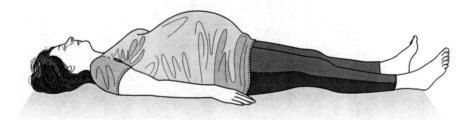

Figure A3.1 Supine position/lying on your back. From the supine position (or from the Trendelenburg position) roll over into the lateral position with the knees bent up towards the abdomen and chest.

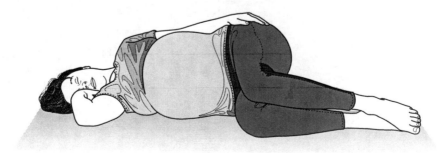

Figure A3.2 Lateral position/lying on your side. *'Please would you roll over on to your side.'*

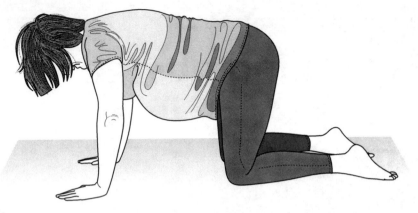

Figure A3.3 Knees and palm position/hands and knees. *'Please would you roll further on to your knees.' 'Now would you lift your shoulders so that you are supporting your weight with your palms and knees.'*

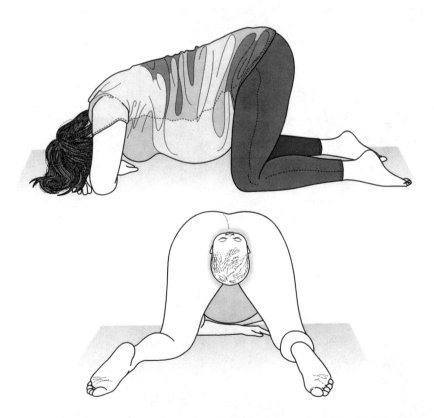

Figures A3.4 & A3.5 Forearm and knees position. Here the woman's head and chest are in a lower plane to that of her buttocks. *'Please now bend your elbows and lean forward so your head is on your forearms.'* The aim of this tilt is to allow for the release of pressure on the prolapsed cord (reverse Trendelenburg).

Appendix 4 – Examples of strategies for communication partners of people with aphasia

From Simmons-Mackie, N., 2001. Social approaches to aphasia intervention. In: Chapey, R. Ed., *Language Intervention Strategies in Aphasia and Related Neurogenic Communication Disorders*, 4th edn. Lippincott, Williams and Wilkins, Philadelphia, p. 276. (Reproduced with kind permission of Lippincott, Williams and Wilkins.)

- Slow the rate of speech
- Chunk ideas with pauses
- Insert pauses between topics
- Simplify sentence structure
- Convey one idea at a time
- Place key information at the end of the sentence
- Repeat key words
- Write key words as referents
- Re-phrase when not understood
- Use direct instead of indirect referents (Mary *vs* she)
- Use gestures, body lean and gaze to shift topics
- Use verbal terminators to end a topic ('so much for that')
- Use verbal introductions to open topics ('Let's talk about')
- Use redundancy ('Where's Spot, the dog? *vs* 'Where's Spot?')
- Use altering phrases or gestures (touch, 'uhh, John')
- Emphasize key content with stress and intonation
- Tolerate silence of the other person
- Use gestures and pantomime to add information while talking
- Backchannel to encourage the aphasic speaker ('I see, oh yes')
- Paraphrase, summarize, or reinterpret to verify, elaborate, and sustain topic
- Verify your understanding by paraphrasing, repeating, or questioning as needed
- Use 'thematic written support' (Garrett and Beukalman 1995)
- Use props (magazines, photo albums, pictures)
- Subtly incorporate words that the person with aphasia 'didn't get' into your own utterances
- Get information from his/her body language – focus on more than the talk
- Progress from general to specific questioning
- Provide and use paper and markers to support talk
- Draw or write key ideas while talking

- Use the augmentative strategies of the person with aphasia to model and establish equality
- Use the environment (talk about a picture on the wall)
- Establish shared experiences as topics (sport, gardening)
- Focus on doing things together versus carrying out discussions

- Avoid teaching comments 'you said that right'
- Reflect feelings communicated non-verbally ('Oh boy, that makes you angry')
- Establish equality in relationship by following the aphasic individual's lead; acknowledge opinions, etc.

Index

Note: Page numbers followed by *f* indicate figures; *b* indicate boxes.